The GP Registrar Survival Guide

Wendy Abrams
(MB BS MRCGP DRCOG)
General Practitioner, London

and

Siân Howell
(MB BS MRCGP DRCOG)
General Practitioner, London

© BIOS Scientific Publishers Limited, 2002

First published 2002

A CIP catalogue record for this book is available from the British Library.

ISBN 1 85996 034 0

BIOS Scientific Publishers Ltd
9 Newtec Place, Magdalen Road, Oxford OX4 1RE, UK
Tel. +44 (0)1865 726286. Fax +44 (0)1865 246823
World Wide Web home page: http://www.bios.co.uk/

Important Note from the Publisher
The Information contained within this book was obtained by BIOS Scientific Publishers Ltd from sources believed by us to be reliable. However, while every effort has been made to ensure its accuracy, no responsibility for loss or injury whatsoever occasioned to any person acting or refraining from action as a result of information contained herein can be accepted by the authors or publishers.

The reader should remember that medicine is a constantly evolving science and while the authors and publishers have ensured that all dosages, applications and practices are based on current indications, there may be specific practices which differ between communities. You should always follow the guidelines laid down by the manufacturers of specific products and the relevant authorities in the country in which you are practising.

Production Editor: Aimie Haylings
Typeset by Saxon Graphics Ltd, Derby, UK
Printed by TJ International Ltd, Padstow, UK

Contents

Abbreviations

A&E	Accident and Emergency
AA	Attendance Allowance
ADR	Adverse drug reaction
AIDS	Acquired Immune Deficiency Syndrome
ALS	Advanced life support
ASW	Approved Social Worker
ATLS	Advanced trauma life support
b.d.	Twice a day
BJGP	*British Journal of General Practice*
BM Stix	Blood glucose monitoring sticks
BMA	British Medical Association
BMI	Body mass index
BMJ	*British Medical Journal*
BNF	*British National Formulary*
BP	Blood pressure
BPA	Basic Practice Allowance
BUPA	British United Provident Association
CD	Controlled drug
CHI	Commission for Health Improvement
CHS	Child Health Surveillance
COC	Combined oral contraceptive pill
CPN	Community psychiatric nurse
CPR	Cardio-pulmonary resuscitation
CRP	C-reactive protein
CXR	Chest X-ray
COPMED	Conference of Postgraduate Medical Deans of the UK
COGPED	Committee of General Practice Education Directors
CV	Curriculum vitae
DCH	Diploma in Child Health
DF 118	Dihydrocodeine tartrate
DFFP	Diploma of the Faculty of Family Planning
DGM	Diploma in Geriatric Medicine
DLA	Disability Living Allowance
DMR	Diploma in Medical Rehabilitation

DN	District nurse
DOH	Department of Health
DPGPE	Director of Postgraduate General Practice Education
DPTC	Disabled Person's Tax Credit
DRCOG	Diploma of the Royal College of Obstetricians and Gynaecologists
DTB	*Drug and Therapeutics Bulletin*
DTMH	Diploma in Tropical Medicine and Hygiene
DVLA	Driver and Vehicle Licensing Agency
DVT	Deep vein thrombosis
DWP	Department for Work and Pensions
eBNF	Electronic British National Formulary
ECG	Electrocardiogram
ENT	Ear, nose and throat
ESR	Erythrocyte sedimentation rate
FBC	Full blood count
FRCGP	Fellow of the Royal College of General Practitioners
GI	Gastrointestinal
GMC	General Medical Council
GMS	General Medical Services
GP	General practitioner
GPC	General Practitioners Committee
GSL	General sales list (medicines classification)
GTN	Glyceryl trinitrate
HIV	Human immune deficiency (or immunodeficiency) virus
HRT	Hormone replacement therapy
HSE	Health and Safety Executive
HV	Health visitor
IBS	Irritable bowel syndrome
ID	Identity
i.m.	Intramuscular
INR	International normalized ratio
INT	Immediately necessary treatment
IOS	Item of service
IT	Information technology
IUCD	Intrauterine contraceptive device
i.v.	Intravenous
IVP	Intravenous pyelogram
JCPTGP	Joint Committee on Postgraduate Training for General Practice
LMC	Local Medical Committee
LoCIUT	Letter of Competence in Intrauterine Techniques
LSD	Lysergic acid diethylamide
MA	Maternity Allowance
MAP	Membership by assessment of performance (of the RCGP)

MAR	Medical Attendant's Report
MBA	Master of Business Administration
MCQ	Multiple choice question
MDI	Metered dose inhaler
MHA	Mental health assessment
MI	Myocardial infarction
MIMS	*Monthly Index of Medical Specialties*
MRCGP	Member/ship of the Royal College of General Practitioners
MS	Multiple sclerosis
MSc	Master of Science
MSU	Mid-stream urine
MW	Midwife
NANP	National Association of Non-Principals
NICE	National Institute for Clinical Excellence
NIPPI	Northern Ireland Prescribing Prices Information
NPC	National Prescribing Centre
NPMS	National Project Marking Schedule (summative assessment)
NPSA	National Patient Safety Agency
NSAID	Non-steroidal anti-inflammatory drug
o.d.	Daily
o.p.	One standard pack (prescription instructions)
OSCE	Objective structured clinical examination
OT	Occupational therapy/ist
OTC	Over-the-counter
P45	Inland Revenue form documenting personal pay and tax details on leaving employment
PACT	Prescribing Analysis and Cost
PC	Performance criteria (for MRCGP video)
PCA	Personal Capability Assessment
PCC	Primary care centre (also post-coital contraception)
PCG	Primary Care Group
PCT	Primary Care Trust
PEFR	Peak expiratory flow rate
PGEA	Postgraduate Education Allowance
PHCT	Primary Health Care Team
PhD	Doctor of Philosophy
PILs	Patient information leaflets
PMH	Past medical history
PMS	Personal Medical Services
PN	Practice nurse
p.o.	By mouth
PoM	Prescription-only medicine
PPA	Prescription Pricing Authority

p.r.	Rectally
p.r.n.	As required
p.v.	Vaginally
q.d.s.	Four times daily
RCP	Royal College of Physicians
RCGP	Royal College of General Practitioners
RMO	Responsible Medical Officer
RSM	Royal Society of Medicine
RTA	Road traffic accident
s.c.	Subcutaneous/ly
SF	Sugar-free
SHO	Senior house officer
SMP	Statutory Maternity Pay
SOAP	Subjective, objective, assessment, plan (acronym to document consultation in medical records)
SPA	Scottish Prescribing Analysis
SSMG	Sure Start Maternity Grant
SSP	Statutory Sick Pay
SW	Social worker
TCA	To come again
TCB	To come back/to call back
TCI	To come in
t.d.s.	Three times daily
TFT	Thyroid function test
TOP	Termination of pregnancy
UTI	Urinary tract infection
VTR/1 & 2	Statements of satisfactory completion of either GP registrar post (VTR/1) or educationally approved posts for GP training (VTR/2)
VTS	Vocational training scheme

Introduction

This guide aims to help bridge the surprisingly large gap between hospital jobs and primary care. The different ethos, professionals, systems and patient presentations can be overwhelming to the newcomer. You will be on a steep learning curve and the registrar year will be gone before you know it.

Following the chronology of the year, we offer guidance on how to organize yourself and approach all the practical aspects of everyday work, the educational hoops of summative assessment and the MRCGP exam. We also hope to instil good practices that will reduce your likelihood of making errors and receiving complaints, whilst keeping you enthusiastic for the busy and varied job of general practice.

Our advice is distilled from our experience and a wide variety of sources but is not intended to be prescriptive. We have tried to include everything we did not know at the beginning of the registrar year but wish we had!

Use the book to supplement input from your trainer, VTS course, local and practice policies and above all your own experience. Annotate it as you go.

General practice is constantly developing and there are frequent changes in the organization of the NHS, GP training, summative assessment and the MRCGP exam. We include directions on how to access the latest information and will keep the book updated on the BIOS website.

We would be delighted to have your feedback and suggestions so email us at, GPSurvivalGuide@bios.co.uk

Enjoy your year!

Wendy Abrams and Siân Howell (October 2001)

Foreword

The transition from hospital medicine to general practice is marked by a profound change within the doctor who undertakes it. Although increasing attention is paid during the undergraduate years to the importance of people and relationships in clinical practice, the development of a true generalist perspective can only take place during the general practice component of post-graduate training.

Many doctors experience extreme disorientation as they discover that common problems in hospital are uncommon outside, that symptoms and signs have different meanings, that patients may have multiple problems all of which they bring to "their" doctor. Also the degree of access that patients have to their GP with the possibility of continuity but also of dysfunctional relationships, can be a source of stress and unexpected confusion. Although the surprises and good experiences compensate and eventually predominate, all of these changes in clinical practice take place within a different culture which appears less hierarchical, may be business orientated and is closely integrated into the surrounding community. It is no wonder that registrars need a Survival Guide!

This book brings a mixture of practical and personal information and guidance assembled from the perspective of authors who have recently survived the transition themselves. It provides a basis for planning and pacing, but it is also a source of encouragement for those who are encountering difficulties. All general practitioners sometimes need to lock the consulting room door and lie down for a few moments. What a relief to discover that the authors have found that too!

The approach to study and to assessment is clear and will help the reader to assign priorities and focus on achieving the JCPTGP certificate to begin unsupervised practice. The role of the Royal College of General Practitioners and the importance of the MRCGP is discussed, opening one of many perspectives for career development after training is over. The foundations for a sensible and rewarding attitude to practice are set out. But most of all, this guide provides information and advice that will develop along with its reader who should annotate it from personal experience. It is designed to be and should be viewed as a dynamic document that will increase in value the more it is used.

Professor Dame Lesley Southgate
(President RCGP)

Acknowledgements

Thanks to the following for their help with this book: Rachel Abrams, Peter Arlett, Melanie Arnold (Department of Health), Margareth Attwood (National Office for Summative Assessment), Leigh Austin (London Deanery), Susie Barnes, Alex Bass (London Ambulance Service), Kambiz Boomla, Tonia Briffa, Katie Carter (JCPTGP), Ruth Clarke, Philippa Cockman, Jenny Delaney (GPC), Jane Durston (DVLA), Sarah Egan (RCGP), Richard Fieldhouse (NANP), Derek Gallen (Oxford Deanery), Michael Golding (Camidoc), Emma Hargreaves, Sharon Hart (Drug and Therapeutics Bulletin), Nina Howell, Anthea Lints (London Deanery), Dinesh Mehta (BNF), Hamish Meldrum (GPC), Gerard Panting (Medical Protection Society), Claire Parry, Philip Sawney (Dept. of Work and Pensions), Pat Sharp, Jonathon Sheldon, Brigid Sheppard, Anita Silk (Dept. of Work and Pensions), Saina Tebble (GMC).

Also thanks to Professor Dame Lesley Southgate, President of the Royal College of General Practitioners, for writing the Foreword.

1
General practice training in the UK

INTRODUCTION

General practice training schemes have been around since the 1950s, but it was not until 1982 that the compulsory 3-year vocational training was introduced. GP training is the shortest specialist training in the UK and has the great advantage of recognizing parts of training from other specialties should a career change be considered.

The organization and requirements of GP training are constantly changing. Check that your training plans fulfil the latest national regulations and local stipulations. The key agencies and individuals involved in GP training are outlined in *Box 1.1*.

TRAINING REQUIREMENTS FOR GENERAL PRACTICE

To practise as an unsupervised GP in the NHS you must hold a JCPTGP certificate of 'Prescribed' or 'Equivalent Experience' (see below) which is issued on completion of GP training. Your certificate is essentially your licence to practise and the type depends on the training you have undertaken. Successful completion of all four components of summative assessment is an essential requirement of the training.* Full details are given in the JCPTGP booklet '*A Guide to Certification*', which is updated annually.

* See Chapter 20: Summative assessment.

Prescribed experience

The standard training for UK general practice, after pre-registration house jobs, is a minimum of 3 years, which must include:

- 1 year as a hospital SHO in 'listed' specialties (*Box 1.2*)
- 1 year as a GP registrar
- 1 year either in listed hospital or GP registrar posts (or a combination).

The usual training involves 2 years in approved hospital posts and 12 months as a GP registrar. A maximum of 12 months only in any one of the listed specialties and a maximum of 6 months in a specialty other than those above (in a post that is approved) can count towards the overall training period.

Provided that all 3 years of training are completed in the 7 years prior to your application you can apply for the certificate of prescribed experience. Statements of satisfactory completion (VTR forms) are required for each period of training (see below).

Box 1.1   Agencies and individuals involved in GP training

Joint Committee on Postgraduate Training for General Practice (JCPTGP)

- Independent body set up by the Royal College of General Practitioners and the General Practitioners Committee
- Approves all training posts
- Sets the standards for GP training in the UK
- Issues the JCPTGP certificate on completion of training (see below)

Directors of Postgraduate General Practice Education (DPGPE or Director)

- Also known as Deans
- Organize, monitor and appoint to vocational training posts
- Work from regional postgraduate deaneries
- Accountable to the Department of Health in England and equivalent bodies in other UK countries
- List of current Directors available from the JCPTGP or the Conference of Postgraduate Medical Deans in the UK (COPMED)

Vocational training schemes (VTS)

- Comprehensive 2- or 3-year schemes of approved posts
- Provide the main means of fulfilling the training requirements for general practice

Course organizers

- Practising GPs
- Run the compulsory VTS release course
- Liaise with the Director and GP trainers

GP trainers

- Practising GPs
- Specifically trained and supported
- Work individually with GP registrars as teachers and mentors within a training practice

Equivalent experience

If you have done non-standard training, for example posts abroad or UK posts completed more than 7 years before making your application, you will need to apply for a certificate of equivalent experience. The JCPTGP looks at the educational content and supervision in such posts together with the skills and experience acquired. It expects a good balance of experience relevant to general practice. It may be able to grant retrospective (generally not prospective) approval for overseas posts. Full details are available from them.

ORGANIZATION OF TRAINING

The main way of fulfilling the training requirements for prescribed experience is through a formal VTS organized through the deaneries. Alternatively, you may do your own DIY scheme, or a combination of both VTS and DIY posts, but there will be few opportunities for DIY schemes in the future.

At the start of training the Director allocates each doctor with a national GP training number for use throughout the 3 years. DIY trainees will need to apply to their Director to obtain a number.

Vocational training schemes

These schemes usually involve four 6-month hospital posts in approved specialties and 12 months as a GP registrar in a local training practice, which may be split into two 6-month periods. Shorter schemes may be available for those who have already completed some posts.

These schemes can be great, particularly if you want to stay in one area and avoid job applications every 6 months. The VTS also guarantees a release course (affectionately known as 'play school') and the support of other GPs in training throughout your hospital posts. However some people find these schemes restrictive and get '18 month burnout' after the third job in a row. If this might be you, consider organizing your own scheme so you can take a break if necessary.

DIY schemes

> **Confirm that your individual training plans fulfil JCPTGP requirements by discussing them with your Director, in the first instance, and then the JCPTGP.**

You can organize your own scheme with jobs of your choice around the country, but you must ensure you fulfil the criteria for prescribed experience. Training in this way provides more flexibility, but also means more frequent job applications and job insecurity.

If you have already completed some posts, or are planning a change of career into general practice, find out how much is already recognized and what you need to do to complete your training.

Innovative (hybrid) schemes

There are an increasing number of innovative or 'hybrid' training schemes on offer, which involve a longer time in general practice (e.g. 18 months) and less time in hospital posts. Some may offer short bursts in GP-relevant specialties such as ENT, dermatology or rheumatology. Other schemes may offer academic placements linked to medical school Departments of General Practice. Provisions vary from region to region so enquire locally. All posts must comply with JCPTGP requirements.

Flexible (part-time) training

GP training can be undertaken part-time and VTS schemes should offer this option. Flexible training should involve no less than 60% of whole-time training (40 months in hospital posts and 20 months in general practice) and be completed within 7 years. This may be reduced to 50% of whole time in the near future in line with flexible training in other specialties. The training must include at least 1 week of full-time work in both hospital and GP posts. Full-time trainees should be able to change to part-time at any stage of their training.

Work and pay of a flexible trainee should represent a pro rata share of the work of a full-timer and also allow for the VTS release course.

Priority for flexible training tends to go to those who would be unable to train at all if they had to train full-time (rather than those combining careers). Organizing flexible training may be difficult so you need to prepare well in advance and discuss your options with your Director. Part-time GP registrar posts are usually easier to organize than hospital posts given that GP registrars are supernumerary.

Non-UK nationals

Doctors who qualified or trained outside the UK, either in the European Economic Area or overseas, may be eligible to undertake GP training, but will need to confirm their ability to work in the UK and GMC registration status and will need to contact the JCPTGP.

Refresher training

Funding may be available, via the Director, for supervised and supported GP posts for GP-trained doctors returning to general practice after a break (e.g. bringing up a family or working abroad) or those who have no experience of working in the NHS.

Extended training

Some regions may offer senior registrar posts for those wishing to gain more supervised experience after successful completion of their GP training.

Registrars who have experienced difficulty completing their training, or passing summative assessment, can apply for an extension of their basic GP training either informally to the Director or formally to the JCPTGP.

APPLYING FOR GP TRAINING

This will depend on whether you undertake a formal VTS or go it alone. The Directors coordinate recruitment to formal VTS schemes and all stand-alone GP registrar posts. This should ensure equal opportunities in interview and appointment procedures and that local needs are met.

VTS

Looking for jobs

Vocational training schemes are advertised together twice a year in the *British Medical Journal* (*BMJ*). Details of all regional schemes are available on the website www.vtsonline.co.uk, a national VTS directory.

For schemes you are interested in request the VTS information pack from the deanery and talk to the course organizers and current GPs in training. Find out:

- what the hospital posts really involve and the level of supervision available
- the choices available for different jobs
- whether there are any innovative schemes on offer
- the low-down on particularly good or bad jobs and training practices
- the summative assessment and MRCGP exam pass rates
- which courses are on offer throughout the scheme.

Your application

Application to most schemes is by application form rather than curriculum vitae, so take time to complete this and do yourself justice. You may apply to more than one deanery but you will need to let each know where you have applied.

Keep abreast of the recent developments in primary care. Clarify why you want to do general practice training. Is it for its own sake or as a stepping-stone to another career such as public health or working abroad?

Hospital jobs

> **Get your VTR/2 forms signed after each post.**

Non-VTS trainees should apply directly to the hospital or trust for individual jobs, which should be approved for GP training before you apply.

Approval of posts

The JCPTGP approves posts that have been approved by their own specialty royal college as suitable for specialist training, then selected by the RCGP and local deanery committees as suitable for general practice training. There are basic criteria that all such posts should fulfil (*Box 1.3*). The RCGP also publishes joint Vocational Training Statements, in conjunction with the other specialty colleges, giving guidance on GP training within hospital posts. These booklets are available from the RCGP, free to GP registrars.*

* See Sources and further reading.

Box 1.3 JCPTGP standards for selection of GP training hospital posts

Posts should have:

- induction course
- named educational supervisor
- written educational aims (based on joint college statements)
- regular assessment of educational needs and educational plan
- appraisal at end of post
- minimum 4 hours protected teaching time
- protected time for VTS release and/or specialty teaching programme
- funding and study leave available for GP-relevant study
- access to postgraduate library and education facilities
- appraisal visit from a course organizer to review progress and troubleshoot
- good balance of service and educational needs
- clinical audit in place
- satisfactory catering and accommodation facilities.

(Not all criteria may be achievable in non-VTS SHO posts.)

Making the most of your hospital posts

As many general practice training-approved hospital posts are still geared to service commitment and specialty training rather than general practice, the onus is on you to be assertive to get the most from the job. Think ahead for GP-relevant experience and skills you should gain from each post and discuss these with your consultant.

If you feel any job has not met your training needs you should let the JCPTGP and your Director know. They can reassess the post, make recommendations and even withdraw approval for GP training.

The registrar year

The GP registrar year does not have to be done in its entirety after your hospital jobs, although the last phase of your training should be as a GP registrar, partly because this will maximize your chances of passing summative assessment. If in your first few months in a practice you feel that you are in the wrong place, or do not get on with your trainer, consider moving for the second 6 months.

Applying for posts

> **Application for all GP registrar posts is through the DPGPE for VTS and DIY trainees.**

Whether you are a VTS or DIY trainee you should have plenty of opportunity to research and state your preferences for a particular practice or trainer, but you cannot apply directly to a practice. Plan ahead, especially if there is a particular practice you have your eye on.

For DIY trainees deaneries will advertise stand-alone GP registrar jobs alongside the VTS posts in the *BMJ*. The Director will also have a list of all local training practices. Bear in mind that you may be competing with VTS colleagues who will have had longer to research the practices and express their preferences. When you apply, send a hand-written covering letter that should explain gaps between jobs and reasons for any relocation.

You are eligible for travel reimbursements for attending interviews so keep receipts.*

* See Allowances and reimbursements, pp. 59 & 60.

Choosing your practice

All trainers and training practices have to fulfil requirements set regionally (*Box 1.4*) which take into account JCPTGP national guidelines. Practices vary widely in their general ethos, organization, finances and attitude to the registrar so take these factors into account when making your choices (*Box 1.5*). Probably the most important factors in choosing a practice are the personality of the trainer and the practice reputation amongst former registrars.

Benefits to the trainer and training practice

Despite the increased workload involved in supervision and tutorials, training practices gain a lot from having a registrar (*Box 1.6*).

DOCUMENTATION FOR THE JCPTGP CERTIFICATE

VTR forms

These 'Statements of Satisfactory Completion' (*Box 1.7*) must be signed after each approved hospital job and GP registrar post, and

Box 1.4 Training practice and trainer requirements

(Reproduced from the London Deanery criteria)

Practice premises
- Adequate premises for list size and in reasonable decorative order
- Sufficient consulting rooms for trainer and registrar to consult at the same time
- Ideally own consulting room for GP registrar
- Common room or library for meetings and tutorials

Equipment and systems
- Computerized, with use during consultation
- Medical records filed in date order
- Drug list and clinical summary in written or computer notes
- Age–sex registers (for immunizations, smears, over-75s checks)
- Reasonable waiting time for appointments and good access for emergencies
- Adequate medical equipment for GP registrar

Staffing
- Sufficient staff, with job descriptions and contracts, adequate training and clear lines of responsibility
- Observable good teamwork practices, regular meetings

Trainer requirements
- Possession of MRCGP (obligatory for new trainers)
- Attendance at introductory trainer's course then refresher course
- Preparation for practice visit and interview including: prepared outline of training programme for the year; written library list; GP registrar assessment procedures; details of previous GP registrar study leave; GP registrar contract; practice report; visit to and report on other training practice(s)
- Enthusiasm for teaching and knowledge of teaching skills, methods and organization
- High standard of patient care and services

Box 1.5   Choosing a practice: checklist

Speak to
- Current registrar
- Trainer
- Practice manager and arrange a visit

Practice profile
- Number of partners and other employed doctors
- List size
- Location: rural, inner city, urban; can you get there easily? will you see your patients in the supermarket?
- Average surgery length, consultation length, number of patients seen
- Range of services offered
- Special interests of partners
- Academic links
- Look at the practice leaflet

Trainer profile
- Gender (is this relevant or not to you?)
- Personality (very important)
- Number of sessions undertaken, overlap with GP registrar sessions
- Reputation as a trainer
- Outside interests

Training set-up
- Are there other registrars in the practice at the same time?
- Your timetable and protected time
- Tutorial time
- Will you have your own room?
- On-call requirements in and out of hours

forwarded with your application for your final certificate (see below). They can be signed in the final 4 weeks of a post and no earlier. Copies of both VTR forms can be downloaded from the JCPTGP website. The forms must be completed accurately otherwise processing your final certificate will be delayed.

Applying for your JCPTGP certificate

You can apply for your certificate in the final 4 weeks of your GP registrar year. Remember that you must have it before you can work in

Box 1.6   Benefits of having a GP registrar

Workload and financial benefits
- Practice receives annual training grant
- Most registrars take on a significant clinical workload as the year progresses
- Registrar audit can help fulfil requirements for clinical governance
- Past registrars are a great pool for locums, assistants and potential partners

Educational and motivational benefits
- Registrars bring useful clinical updates from recent hospital experience
- Give fresh viewpoints on old practice habits
- Teaching provides stimulation
- Trainers are kept 'on their toes', preventing burnout

Box 1.7   VTR forms

VTR/2
- Covers hospital posts
- Must be signed by supervising consultant and Director of the region where post undertaken
- Must bear hospital and trust stamp
- Held by medical staffing

VTR/1
- Covers GP registrar post(s)
- Must be signed by GP trainer and endorsed by your Director
- Director must also confirm successful completion of summative assessment
- Separate forms required for each period as GP registrar even if with same trainer

Box 1.8   Checklist for JCPTGP certificate application

(Keep photocopies of everything)

Prescribed experience
- Letter with name, address and GMC number
- GMC certificate or photocopy
- Original VTR/2 forms for each hospital post completed accurately (*Box 1.7*)
- Original VTR/1 forms signed by your trainer and Director

Equivalent experience
- As above, plus:
  - Specific application form
  - Additional forms from JCPTGP for overseas posts or those undertaken more than 7 years previously

Send to
- The Joint Honorary Secretaries, The Joint Committee on Postgraduate Training for General Practice, 14 Princes Gate, Hyde Park, London SW7 1PU

---

any capacity as an unsupervised GP. Minor inaccuracies on the forms are a common cause of delay in processing your certificate, so be ready to apply as early as possible. You will need the 4 weeks to iron out any problems.

Application is by letter for the certificate of prescribed experience and by form for equivalent experience (available from the JCPTGP). Include all the necessary paperwork (*Box 1.8*). Ensure that any part-time posts clearly indicate the percentage of full-time commitment and that all dates are accurate, with no overlapping periods or gaps on the same certificate. Stipulate the precise dates of any maternity, sick or unpaid leave.

Certificates of prescribed experience should be issued within 2 weeks of application, but those for equivalent experience may take at least 8 weeks for processing.

SOURCES AND FURTHER READING

1. Department of Health, *The GP Registrar Scheme, Vocational Training for General Medical Practice, The UK Guide*, April 2000; www.doh.gov.uk/pdfs/gpmanual.pdf

2. JCPTGP, *A Guide to Certification*, 2001; www.jcptgp.org.uk
3. JCPTGP, *The Selection of Hospital Posts for General Practice Training*, 2001.
4. JCPTGP, *Recommendations on the Selection of General Practice Trainers*, 2001.
5. RCGP and specialty college Joint Vocational Statements:
- RCGP and Royal College of Obstetricians and Gynaecologists, *General Practitioner Vocational Training in Obstetrics and Gynaecology*, 1998.
- RCGP and Royal College of Paediatrics and Child Health, *The Paediatric Component of Vocational Training for General Practice*, 1998.
- RCGP and British Association of A&E Medicine, *General Practitioner Vocational Training in Accident and Emergency Medicine*, 1998.
- RCGP, *The Quality of Hospital-based Education for General Practice*, 1998.
- RCGP and Royal College of Psychiatrists, *General Practitioner Vocational Training in Psychiatry*, 1998.
- RCGP and Association for Palliative Medicine, *Palliative Medicine Content of Vocational Training for General Practice*, 1998.
- RCGP and the British Association of Dermatologists, *Dermatology for General Practice Trainees*, 1998.
- RCGP and the Royal College of Ophthalmologists, *Ophthalmology for General Practice Trainees*, 2001.
- RCGP and British Geriatric Society, *General Practitioner Vocational Training in Geriatric Medicine*, 1998.
6. BMA General Practitioners Committee, *GP Registrars' Pack*, May 2001.
7. BMA General Practitioners Committee, *Guidance for GP Registrars*, November 1999.
8. Field S. *Vocational Training for General Practice*, Careers Focus, *BMJ* (Classified) 2000; 19/26 August, 2–3.
9. Conference of Postgraduate Medical Deans in the UK; www.copmed.org.uk

2
The GP and how general practice works

INTRODUCTION

Despite the ever-changing and increasing role of the GP in the UK, the main *raison d'être* has changed little over the last 50 years. General practice within the NHS provides direct personal and family health services to a small community over many years.

The GP is one of the first ports of entry into the NHS and has a gate-keeper and coordination role for secondary care and other services. GPs deal with new problems, chronic illnesses, emergency medical care as well as health promotion and the particular health needs of their community.

There are over 38 000 GPs working in the UK as both principals and non-principals (see below). Over the last 10 years there has been a significant increase in the percentage of non-principals. Most GPs work in partnerships with the number of single-handed GPs decreasing. An estimated 98% of the UK population is registered with a GP.

TYPES OF GP

Broadly speaking GPs are classified as either principals or non-principals (*Box 2.1*). A principal has a contract held by the health authority to take unsupervised responsibility for a list of patients. They may work full or part-time. 'Principal' and 'partner' are often used synonymously, although not all principals work in partnership. Most partnerships work within the framework of a legally binding 'partnership agreement'.

Non-principals do not have a direct contract with the health authority but are generally employed and paid by a practice, or sometimes by a Primary Care Group (PCG) or Primary Care Trust (PCT) or equivalent body in Scotland or Wales.

GP CONTRACT

Most GP principals are self-employed and have a contract with the health authority to provide services to patients. This contract can be through GMS* or the more recently introduced PMS.†

The GMS contract is outlined in the 'Terms of Service' and the rates and conditions of remuneration are detailed in the *Statement of Fees and Allowances* (The Red Book) which is a complex, nationally nego-tiated set of terms and conditions for general practice work (*Box 2.2*). The GMS contract is held by the health authority on behalf of the Secretary of State and GPs are paid by the health authority for providing GMS services to patients. These payments are used to cover

* General Medical Services.
† Personal Medical Services.

Box 2.1 Types of GP

GP principals

Unrestricted principal
- Provides a full range of General Medical Services (GMS) or Personal Medical Services (PMS)
- List not limited to any particular group of patients
- Self-employed
- Contract held by health authority

Restricted principal

Provides *either*:
- A full range of GMS/PMS to a limited group of patients *or*
- specific services only (such as maternity)

Salaried partner
- Partnership status but with a guaranteed salaried income rather than a share of practice profits

Non-principals

GP assistants
- Employed by a practice to help with clinical workload

GP associates (of which there are very few)
- Work *either* for a single-handed, isolated or group of practices *or*
- With a particular arrangement with a health authority

GP locums
- Employed by practices to cover leave and other absence
- Work on a short-term or occasional basis
- Usually paid on a sessional basis
- Self-employed

GP retainers
- Work a minimum one session a week and maximum of 52 sessions a quarter due to outside commitments, such as childcare
- Part of salary reimbursed by the health authority
- Employing GPs responsible for continued training and support
- Posts usually restricted to 5 years duration

Box 2.2 Some stipulations of GP Terms of Service for GMS

Practice population and premises
- List size
- Type of each patient on list – permanent or temporary and for how long
- Stipulations for practice area and boundaries
- Standards for practice premises

Services provided
- Services provided – 'all necessary and appropriate medical services of the type usually provided by GPs'
- Optional services (maternity, contraception, child health surveillance, minor surgery) with training requirements and fees payable
- Fees for services provided
- Registration health assessment for newly registered patients
- Practice leaflet for patients with specified information

Staffing
- GP availability – minimum hours available to patients stipulated for full and part-time principals
- Acceptable cover for GP absences, use of deputies and out-of-hours cover
- Employees – staffing levels for which partial reimbursement is available

Others
- Standards for medical records
- Requirement to notify health authority of change of GP residence
- Requirement for Annual Practice Report
- Information for Local Directory of Principals

building, staffing, computer and other costs and the individual GPs' income. Most partners take a monthly drawing and may receive an extra payment at the end of the financial year if their share of the total yearly profits exceeds their drawings.

PMS contracts, on the other hand, are negotiated locally between individual GPs or practices and the health authority or PCT. They have been introduced in an attempt to reduce the administrative burden of making claims via GMS and also to allow GPs to develop services appropriate to local need.

GP INCOME

The self-employed GP principal derives income from both NHS and non-NHS sources.

NHS income

Fees for services are stipulated in The Red Book for GMS (*Box 2.3*) or in individual contracts for PMS. Item of service (IOS) fees are only paid if the practice claims for them, so much effort is put into developing efficient practice systems for claims. As a GP registrar you will be involved in providing and claiming for some of these services.*

* See also Practice systems, p. 49.

Box 2.3   NHS allowances and fees for General Medical Services

Practice population-related
- Basic Practice Allowance (BPA) linked to availability
- Capitation fee – payment per patient, higher for those over 65 and 75
- Deprivation payments – for working in an area of designated deprivation

GP-related
- Postgraduate Education Allowance (PGEA) for attending designated number of hours of education on: disease management; service management; health promotion topics.
- Seniority payments – payable after 7 years as a GP, increasing with time

Patient service-related
- Chronic disease management (such as diabetes and asthma)
- IOS fees – emergency treatment, immediately necessary treatment (INT); night visits; contraceptive services and IUCD insertions; obstetric care; child health surveillance; minor surgery; some childhood immunizations; some foreign travel vaccinations
- Target-based – cervical cytology; most childhood immunizations
- Sustained quality allowance

Reimbursements/grants
- Proportion of staff salaries and pension contributions
- Rent and some other buildings charges
- Computer systems
- Premises improvement grants
- Training grants for GP registrars

Many computerized practices are linked directly with the health authority and a specific computer entry automatically results in an IOS claim.* PMS contracts should relieve practices of the need to make many individual claims, but there are other conditions applied to them.

* See Links, p. 122.

Non-NHS income

GPs may also provide a number of services that are not provided by the NHS, and so are not reimbursed (*Box 2.4*). They are not obliged to provide these services, but if they agree to do so they can charge a fee. Such fees may be charged either to the patient or the third party requesting the GP service, e.g. a medical examination for insurance purposes.†

† See Charging for extras, p. 159.

Box 2.4   Non-NHS fees

GP services within the practice
- Fee payable by patient:
  - some travel vaccinations
  - full medical examination, e.g. for HGV licence, pre-employment, fitness to drive
  - private sick note (ideally employer should pay)
  - fitness to travel certificate
  - holiday cancellation letter
  - completion of private health insurance claim forms
  - statement of fact, e.g. confirmation of address
  - passport/driving licence photo confirmation
  - vaccination certificate
  - freedom from infection certificate.
- Fee payable by requesting organization:
  - medical attendant's reports (for life assurance/mortgage purposes)
  - police reports
  - legal reports
  - cremation forms
  - disabled parking badge
  - taxi card.

Other work within the practice
- Medical student teaching
- Private patients (include tourists and non-UK nationals ineligible for NHS care)

Work undertaken outside the practice
- Police surgeon
- Community clinical medical officer
- Hospital clinical assistantships
- Private screening medicals

GPs may also supplement their income with work outside of the practice, so long as they fulfil their contracted hours of availability to patients and have the agreement of their partners. Non-NHS income may be pooled as general income for the practice or kept by the individual GP.

HOW THE PRACTICE IS ORGANIZED

GP principals essentially run their own small businesses and so have great flexibility in how they organize themselves, their premises and the services they offer. Each practice and each GP will have variable working patterns, which develop over time and change to meet the needs of doctors, staff and patients. We touch on a few of these elements here, and also in Section D, Day-to-day Clinical Work of the GP Registrar.

Running the practice

GP principals have the financial, management and staffing responsibilities of running a business but usually little or no formal training in business or management skills. They are also responsible for maintaining their surgery premises, which may be owned or leased. While some GPs feel these responsibilities conflict with the basics of providing medical care, others like the control over their own working environment.

During the year GP registrars can get a feel for what is involved in running a practice, particularly if you are considering becoming a partner in the future.

The working day

Some practices start with commuter surgeries at 7 a.m., while others may have a later start and/or late evening surgeries. Some practices will close to patients completely between morning and evening surgery, with access to the doctor only in emergencies. Larger practices may be more flexible in their opening hours and the services they provide, but may offer a less personalized service than smaller practices.

Appointments

Appointment types and systems vary, but there are a few main types (*Box 2.5*) and there is no ideal appointments system.

The wait for a routine appointment varies between GPs, practices and with the time of year, but there should always be same-day access for emergencies. Practices should try to offer appointments with the patient's choice of doctor within a few days, but in reality this may be over a week, which causes considerable stress for patients, staff and doctors, may lead to overbooked emergency clinics.

Staff should not overbook your surgeries, but if they need to, it should only be with your permission. You may occasionally want to book an extra appointment into your surgery yourself.

Some practices hold back appointments for the following day, or appointments that can only be made by the doctors. If you have a patient who often takes longer than their appointment allows or has a new problem that will take some time to sort out, you could ask them to book a double appointment or the last appointment of the day.

Box 2.5   Appointment types

Routine
- Usually booked in advance with the patient's registered or preferred GP
- Vary from 5 to 15 minutes
- For non-emergency problems, management of chronic illness or ongoing problems

Emergency
- Usually available on the day, or at short notice
- Short appointments for problems that cannot wait for a routine appointment

Walk-in
- Patients seen on a 'first come, first served' basis

Personal lists

The health authority registers each patient under a particular partner's name. Some practices enforce these 'personal lists' with only the registered doctor seeing their own patients for routine and emergency appointments and home visits. This improves continuity for the patient, but gives them little choice should they wish to change their GP within the practice. Other practices will allow patients to choose which GP they wish to see and encourage them to then stick to that GP, irrespective of their registered GP. Some practices have a more relaxed attitude and allow patients to see whichever GP they wish, or is available at the time.

As a GP registrar you will often see new patients, those who do not have an established relationship with a partner, or those who can simply get an appointment with you sooner than with their usual doctor.*

* See Your case mix, p. 83.

SOURCES AND FURTHER READING

1. Fry J. *General Practice – The Facts.* Radcliffe Medical Press, 1993.
2. Ellis N., Chisholm J. *Making Sense of the Red Book.* 3rd edn. Radcliffe Medical Press, 1997.
3. RCGP Information Sheet no. 1. *Profile of UK General Practitioners.* November 2000.
4. Department of Health; www.doh.gov.uk

3
Other professionals working in primary care

INTRODUCTION

As a GP you will work alongside many other professionals in the community. An understanding of the training, skills and remit of these colleagues will help you refer to them appropriately and optimize care for your patients.

These professionals are employed by different community agencies (GPs, community trusts, PCTs and the local authority) and this can be confusing to the newcomer. They may cover different catchment areas from your practice area and from each other.

This chapter gives an overview of the remit of these colleagues, but you will need to find out their precise roles within your practice.

THE PRIMARY HEALTH CARE TEAM (PHCT)

This embodies the clinical and administrative staff (*Box 3.1*) working together for the care of a practice population.

Box 3.1   The core Primary Health Care Team

- GPs
- Practice nurses
- District nurses
- Health visitors
- Practice manager
- Administrative staff

In your induction period you should have opportunity to accompany some of these professionals and to find out how best to use their services.*

* See Practice staff, pp. 47 & 49.

GP principals directly employ clinical and administrative in-house staff whereas community and primary care trusts employ community medical staff (mainly district nurses, health visitors and midwives). These may be based in your surgery premises but 'shared' with other practices.

Although each professional retains individual responsibility and accountability for their work the GP often assumes leadership of the team. This can sometimes be inappropriate, especially where other team members are more skilled to lead on a particular issue or patient. The GP does, however, retain overall clinical responsibility for the patient.

STAFF EMPLOYED BY GP PRINCIPALS

Nursing staff

Practice nurse

Most practices will employ a practice nurse, who may hold a practice nurse diploma. Their role varies between practices (*Box 3.2*), depending on their training and confidence, and the degree of responsibility given by the partners. GP principals retain responsibility for their training and supervision, as well as for their clinical work and decisions.

Much of the practice nurse work is essential for generating practice income, either for IOS fees or for reaching targets.

Develop a close working relationship with your nurse and make yourself available to give clinical advice and support. Hopefully they

---

Box 3.2   Tasks within the practice nurse remit

Health checks
- New patient registration checks
- Asthma and diabetic clinics
- Elderly health checks

Practical procedures
- Blood pressure measurement
- Blood tests
- Dressing and wound care
- Spirometry
- Cervical smears
- Suture removal
- Immunizations
- Ear syringing
- Cap fitting

Health promotion
- Contraception
- Diet
- Exercise
- Smoking cessation
- Alcohol consumption
- Sexual health
- Travel advice

---

will be mutually obliging and help you out with nursing tasks on your patients that arise during your surgeries.

Nurse practitioner

Nurse practitioners work with, rather than for, GPs and may be employed together with a practice nurse. They all hold the Royal College of Nursing Nurse Practitioner degree. Nurse practitioners take on more responsibility than practice nurses, with an obvious overlap in roles. They have a limited role in prescribing, give telephone advice and undertake home visits. They may triage emergency cases and see uncomplicated presentations in the surgery. Some GP cooperatives and surgeries employ nurse practitioners to provide the first clinical contact with patients.*

* See GP Cooperatives, p. 177.

Administrative staff

Practice manager

The practice manager is responsible for the overall running of the practice. They manage the staff and practice finances, oversee day-to-day administration, liaise with outside agencies and deal with any problems arising. An experienced, senior practice manager may take the practice lead on audit, clinical governance and forward planning. Your practice manager will organize your pay, pension, contract and leave.†

† See Chapter 6: The GP registrar contract and finances.

There are diplomas in practice management and many regions run part-time local training, although these are not mandatory. Practice managers come from a variety of career backgrounds including management or nursing.

Receptionists

Good receptionists are the backbone of a good practice. Their remit includes dealing with patient requests, appointments, prescriptions and medical records as well as other administrative tasks as required by the practice. They should *never* give clinical advice. Although courses exist, most will have no particular training for what can be a complex and stressful job.

Long-serving receptionists can be a mine of useful information on the who's who of patients, including the local 'celebrities'.

Remember that they are on the front line and often take a lot of grief from patients. Support them by reinforcing to patients the practice policies on the use of emergency appointments, requests for repeat prescriptions, etc., particularly where you know patients have been difficult at reception. If a patient has been rude to a receptionist then ask them to apologize directly.

Secretary

Most practices have full or part-time secretaries who type referral letters, arrange faxes, chase up appointments and may deal with other administrative or IT tasks.

They may have a thorough knowledge of local consultants, private specialists, agencies and waiting times.

Other administrative staff

Practices may employ administrators to assist the practice manager, clerks (for filing, photocopying, ordering leaflets, general office duties) and staff with IT skill for inputting clinical information, organizing searches and audit.

Cleaners

Cleaners may come in daily and may have a responsibility for locking up the surgery at the end of the day.

Temporary staff

Additional staff may be employed temporarily, such as medical students to summarize medical records or other staff when major administrative changes are under way.

COMMUNITY CLINICAL TEAM

District nurses

District nurses, also known as community nurses, have a community nursing qualification and are involved mainly in the care of the housebound. They are particularly skilled in the management of long-term disability and chronic illness (*Box 3.3*), but do not provide personal care such as washing, dressing and feeding.

Liaise with district nurses before and after visiting any housebound patients they know.* It is good practice to write a short entry in a patient's district nursing record, usually left at the patient's home, particularly if management changes are needed. You should also communicate changes directly to the nursing team.

* See An approach to visiting, pp. 171–173.

Practices should hold regular meetings with the district nurse team to review and revise management plans for shared patients.

Health visitors

Health visitors are responsible for health promotion and prevention, working with individuals, families and groups. They are trained

Box 3.3   Tasks within the district nurse
              remit

- Ulcer and wound care
- Ensuring drug compliance
- Continence assessments and organizing pads, catheter care and commodes
- Phlebotomy (on patients under their care)
- Monitoring some chronic diseases
- Palliative care

nurses with a health visitor's certificate and are often also midwifery-trained.

The majority of their work is with children aged 10 days to 5 years and a good health visitor is a mine of useful information on childcare and rearing.

They undertake much of the child development and screening work and monitor families at risk. They can provide support to families who are having difficulties coping.*

* See also Child protection, p. 239.

Community midwives

Community midwives see women for antenatal care in the community, either in clinics or at the woman's home, and liaise with the GP and hospital obstetricians involved in the woman's shared care. They can work independently in uncomplicated cases, but must request a doctor's opinion when complications arise.

They have a major role in home births (more so than many GPs) and also aim to attend women in hospital during labour whom they have seen in the community. They will visit mothers and babies at home regularly for the first 10 days after delivery, after which the health visitor takes over.

If your training practice does not have a midwife-led clinic, find out where they take place locally and ask to sit in.

Community physiotherapists

Community physiotherapists provide physiotherapy to housebound patients. Their remit includes therapy for stroke patients cared for at home (and these require an urgent GP referral), assessments for those with acute and disabling back pain and management of chronic chest cases and falls.

They can help to avoid admissions and may alert you when they feel a rheumatological or orthopaedic opinion is needed.

They may also work with paediatric home-care teams, providing regular or intermittent input to children needing mobility, stretching and chest physiotherapy.

Community psychiatric nurses

Community psychiatric nurses (CPNs) work with psychiatrists, mental health social workers and GPs in the care of patients with chronic mental health problems in the community. Although all such patients should have a named CPN, in many areas the service is very stretched.

CPNs will accept new GP referrals and assess patients in their homes or at a community clinic. They see their clients regularly for support and counselling, which can be increased when needed. They will advise you of new problems and when they feel medication changes are appropriate. They may be able to avert admissions or at least inform you, or the psychiatrist, when admission might be required.

Some community mental health teams now provide out-of-hours crisis helplines, manned by CPNs, for known mental health patients who need extra support.

Community paediatric team

Community paediatric teams (*Box 3.4*) work with children with development and speech delay, and behavioural and emotional problems. They may work from purpose-built clinics, and accept referrals from GPs, school nurses and health visitors.

Box 3.4   Community paediatric team

- Community paediatrician
- Physiotherapists
- Occupational therapists
- Speech therapists
- Audiology services
- Psychologists
- Child psychiatrists

---

* See Child protection, p. 239.

Community paediatricians coordinate local services for immunizations, child health surveillance and children with special needs and are available to GPs for advice on such issues. They may be involved in child protection procedures* and often run special immunization clinics for children with egg allergy or previous immunization reactions.

LOCAL AUTHORITY STAFF

Local authorities generally employ the staff involved in social care and housing: social workers, home helps and local authority housing staff and wardens. There can be unclear distinctions as to which services provide personal care, such as washing and dressing, as opposed to nursing care. District nurses will usually make clear to you what is outside their remit.

Social workers

Social workers have a degree or diploma in social work. Within their specialties (below) they have wide-ranging roles, some of which overlap significantly with health professionals. They will take referrals from the clients or their carers as well as from GPs. Their catchment areas may not coincide with your practice, so you may need to be familiar with several offices.

A duty social worker is on-call 24 hours a day for emergencies, mostly relating to mental health sections and child protection. Each specialist team will also have a duty social worker taking the referrals for that day.

Social services for the elderly

Refer your patients to arrange assessments for services (*Box 3.5*).

Box 3.5   Social services for the elderly

- Home help
- Meals-on-wheels
- Personal care
- Night sitters
- Day-centre attendance
- Assessments for possible residential care (local authority or private)

Although many hospital admissions could probably be avoided by increased social care, lack of resources and carers often makes this impossible in practice. Patients requiring 24-hour social care at home may only be offered a maximum three-times-a-day care package, so medical and nursing services may be needed if the patient is not coping.

Mental health social services

Most patients with chronic mental health problems living in the community will have a named social worker, often working in a community mental health team with CPNs. They will help patients with social, benefit and housing needs as well as support and counselling. Approved Social Workers are key players in arranging sections.*

* See The Mental Health Act and the acutely mentally ill patient, p. 250.

Children and families social services

Children and families social workers have a statutory duty to investigate cases where a child is at risk.† There is often both stigma and fear attached to referral to family social services so emphasize their supportive role and the benefit of their early involvement.

† See Child protection, p. 239.

Community occupational therapists

Occupational therapists (OTs) help patients of all ages overcome and live with disability. They have degree level training and may be employed either by health-care trusts (community and hospital) or local authorities.

Hospital OTs generally assess patients prior to discharge and arrange small amendments to the home and appliances, whereas local authority OTs assess individuals already in the community and can arrange more significant changes such as grab rails, ramps and bath aids. Some home amendments are available to all, whether in private, rented or local authority accommodation.

OTHER SESSIONAL WORKERS

A variety of professional and voluntary workers (*Box 3.6*) may do regular or occasional sessions in your practice, particularly if you are based in a large health centre. These include professionals employed by GPs, as well as hospital consultants undertaking community sessions and voluntary sector workers leasing a room. Complementary health services may be offered in-house, although they are rarely NHS-funded. Find out who comes and when so you can make the best use of services on your doorstep.

Box 3.6 Professionals undertaking sessional work in the practice

Health Care
- Counsellors and clinical psychologists
- Hospital consultants
- Physiotherapists
- Occupational therapists
- Specialist nurses, e.g. continence nurse, ulcer nurse, colostomy advisor
- Podiatrist
- Dietician
- Alcohol and drug workers
- Complementary therapists

Social Care
- Citizens' Advice Bureau worker
- Benefits advisor
- Age Concern worker
- Social worker

Counsellors and psychologists

Many practices employ counsellors and psychologists, who may be based in a local psychotherapy or counselling service but undertake sessions at your practice. Discuss individual cases with the counsellor to ensure that you make appropriate referrals, and encourage feedback.

OTHER COMMUNITY HEALTH PROFESSIONALS

All of the following are available on the high street as a private service, but it is useful to know of your local (if limited) NHS community services and who is eligible for referral.

Pharmacists

Pharmacists are highly trained professionals with more knowledge of medication than the average GP will gain in a lifetime. They are often an underused resource. You will have daily interactions with your local pharmacists whenever you write a prescription and there will often be much mutual exchange over patients and prescribing queries.

Your health authority or PCT may employ a pharmacist to advise on local prescribing initiatives and help GPs with audit and evidence-based prescribing.* * See Drug information sources, p. 112.

Podiatrists (chiropodists)

Hospitals, PCTs and community trusts employ podiatrists to provide foot-care services for particular populations (usually the elderly and patients with diabetes) as well as those with other clinical needs such as in-growing toenails, flat feet and bunions. Private high street chiropodists cater for the rest, usually for a reasonable charge.

Opticians

Most high street opticians work privately, but may be contracted to provide certain NHS health services such as diabetic eye screening. They are reimbursed for services provided to patients who are exempt from charges.

Opticians cannot refer directly to an ophthalmologist so when they feel this is necessary they will request a GP referral by forwarding a GOS 18 form. This should be signed by a GP and sent on to the local eye department with the patient's relevant medical history and medication list.

Dentists

Community dentists are usually self-employed but some may work for the PCT or community trust. High street dentists offer a private or NHS service or a combination of the two. They are reimbursed by the health authority for NHS dental care provided to patient groups exempt from charges. There are relatively few NHS dentists, so find out who provides this locally.

All dentists should provide an out-of-hours service to their patients for dental emergencies, so this should not fall to GPs.

GPs are occasionally asked to prescribe prophylactic antibiotics to patients at risk from endocarditis before dental treatment, and for details of medical conditions that may affect their dental treatment. Dentists can prescribe antibiotics themselves.

Hospital dental departments deal with specialist dental needs.

SOURCES AND FURTHER READING

1. RCGP. Information Sheet no. 21. *The Primary Health Care Team.* January 1998.

4
Outside organizations

INTRODUCTION

The work of GPs is affected by the constant organizational change in the NHS. Although changes can appear to be instituted without consultation with the 'shop-floor' workers GPs do have representation that can influence the directives from on high.

As a GP registrar you can get involved through the GP Registrars' Subcommittee of the General Practitioners Committee (GPC) of the British Medical Association (BMA, see below).

It is worth keeping abreast of the changes in health-care organization and medical politics both for your future career and the MRCGP exam.

Although there are many bodies relevant to the GP registrar we have selected here only those you are most likely to hear about or need to contact. We have divided them into professional, service-related, 'political' and educational for clarity and given a brief outline of their remits. Further information is available on their websites.*

* See Sources and further reading.

PROFESSIONAL

General Medical Council

This national regulatory body acts as the watchdog for professional standards for doctors working in the UK. It both sets and oversees standards for medical education and professional practice. The main job of the General Medical Council (GMC) is to protect the public – rather than doctors. It is self-financing through the annual retention fee.

The GMC has four main functions in law:

- to keep up-to-date registers of qualified doctors
- to foster good medical practice
- to promote high standards of medical education
- to deal firmly and fairly with doctors whose fitness to practise is in doubt.

It has the power to remove doctors from the register temporarily or permanently and so remove their right to practise in the UK. You can be removed from the register merely through failing to pay the annual retention fee.

The GMC's advice to doctors on good professional conduct is formalized in its set of guidance booklets '*Duties of a Doctor*', and must be followed as an obligation of registration.† You should receive regular updates of these. Read them and keep for reference and the MRCGP exam.

† See Preventing complaints: keeping yourself informed, p. 221 and Duties of a doctor, p. 224.

NHS-RELATED

Organization of the NHS

The structure and management of the NHS varies between UK countries (*Box 4.1*) and undergoes constant change. See websites* for
national developments.

* See Sources and further
reading.

Box 4.1 Organization of the NHS throughout the UK 2001

National

England	Wales	Scotland	Northern Ireland
The Department of Health	NHS Office of the National Assembly	Scottish Executive Health Department	Department of Health, Social Services and Public Safety
NHS Executive			Health and Social Services Executive
Health Authorities	Health Authorities	Health Boards	Health Boards/ Regional Strategic Authority

Community level

England	Wales	Scotland	Northern Ireland
NHS Trusts – hospital, community and primary care	NHS Trusts – hospital, community and primary care and local health groups	Health Trusts – hospital, community and primary care and local healthcare cooperatives	Health and Social Services Trusts/Health and Social Care Systems

---

At the time of going to press, in England, the Department of Health
works through eight regional NHS Executive offices, which in turn
supervise health authorities. These are responsible for the planning
and quality of health care in their given area. With the advent of
PCTs (see below), the number of health authorities will be reduced
and their role changed. By 2004 the NHS Executive will be
disbanded.

There are some special health authorities that are UK-wide such as transplant services and special hospitals.

Primary Care Groups

These self-governing agencies, introduced in 1999 in England, replaced the existing fund-holders and commissioning groups to allow for greater responsibility for deciding resource allocation to those working closest to patients.

A PCG represents about 50 GPs and between 50 000 and 250 000 patients and works with the health authority to commission services. All PCGs must have become PCTs by 2004.

Primary Care Trusts

PCTs are responsible for both delivery of primary care services and community services and commissioning secondary care services, and are accountable to their health authority.

Quality assurance services

National Institute of Clinical Excellence

This special health authority for England and Wales was set up in 1999 to reduce the inequity of 'postcode' medical care. The National Institute of Clinical Excellence (NICE) produces guidance for use by professionals and the public on health technologies, clinical management of specific conditions, and referrals from primary to secondary care, based on evidence of clinical and cost effectiveness.

NICE guidance is circulated to doctors on a regular basis and is available on their website.

Commission for Health Improvement

This independent commission was set up in April 2000 to improve the quality of health care across England and Wales. It has set up a 4-yearly rolling programme of clinical governance reviews.* The Commission for Health Improvement (CHI) will review all NHS organizations (health authorities, hospitals, PCTs and GP practices), aiming to guarantee the quality of services to patients throughout the NHS. It will also investigate potentially serious service failures.

* See Clinical governance, p. 232.

National Patient Safety Agency

This was set up by the Department of Health in July 2001 as an independent body to improve patient safety by reducing the risk of harm through error.

Its remit is to collect and analyse data on errors, learn lessons and produce solutions for all sectors of the NHS.

New clinical services

NHS Direct

This 24-hour nurse-led telephone service in England and Wales (NHS-24 in Scotland) offers advice on personal health issues and information on accessing NHS services.

It is developing a role in providing out-of-hours care in conjunction with GP services.*

* See Chapter 18: Out-of-hours work, Introduction, p. 176.

Walk-in centres

Introduced in 1999 in various sites in England these centres provide a nurse-led service to 'complement and supplement' GP services. Their remit is to provide face-to-face advice on minor illness and injuries, and health promotion issues. They are open during the day, evenings and weekends. More are planned, but their full impact on GP workload and patient satisfaction has yet to be fully evaluated.

GP POLITICAL

Employers must allow additional paid leave to attend representative meetings, under trade union law. If you are involved you should seek your trainer's approval for such leave.

British Medical Association

As the professional association and union for UK doctors, the BMA lobbies government on issues affecting doctors via its numerous standing committees (see GPC below).

Eighty percent of UK doctors are members. Benefits include the weekly *BMJ*, access to Medline and an excellent library. Advice on working practices, disputes, entitlements and staffing issues are available to members through the regional offices.

General Practitioners Committee (GPC)

As the sole negotiating body for GPs with the Department of Health, this standing committee of the BMA represents all GPs working in the NHS in the UK. Separate Welsh and Scottish committees have been set up with devolution. The Northern Ireland Committee is autonomous of the GPC but works closely with it.

GP Registrars' Subcommittee of the GPC

This represents GPs in training in both hospital and general practice posts. Representatives are elected to the main subcommittee from

* See The GP registrar
contract and finances, p. 53.

regional registrars' committees. It is involved in devising policy nationally and advising on terms of service and educational issues. It produces a newsletter and updated guidance on GP registrars' employment, contract and salary issues.* A list of local representatives and committees is available from the BMA.

Local Medical Committee

The Local Medical Committee (LMC) is a statutory body and is made up of locally elected GPs who meet monthly to discuss and represent GPs' interests and working practices. LMC representatives meet annually at a national conference and approved motions are passed to the GPC for implementation. Each LMC is funded by levies from local GP principals.

National Association of Non-Principals

This association represents some of the estimated 7500 qualified, non-principals or 'independent' GPs in the UK. They aim to ensure representation of non-principals on LMCs and the GPC. The National Association of Non-Principals (NANP) lobbies for employment and pension rights and the inclusion of non-principals in educational initiatives and information distribution. They produce a regular newsletter and put non-principals in touch with each other for local support and study groups.† They have a useful website and handbook available on-line and hold a regular conference. GP registrars can join free of charge.

† See Working as a non-
principal, p. 262.

GP EDUCATIONAL

Directors of Postgraduate General Practice Education

See Chapter 1: General Practice Training in the UK, *Box 1.1*.

Joint Committee on Postgraduate Training for General Practice

See Chapter 1: General Practice Training in the UK, *Box 1.1*.

Royal College of General Practitioners

The Royal College of General Practitioners (RCGP) acts as the voice of GPs on education, training, research and standards. It has 31 faculties throughout the UK that organize educational and social events.

Membership of the college (MRCGP) is either through success in the exam* or by Assessment of Performance (MAP).

* See Chapter 21: The MRCGP Exam

Associate membership is available, at a reduced subscription, to those in training or who do not wish to sit the exam but want to support the college, and all GP registrars are encouraged to join. Fellowship of the college (FRCGP) is by assessment or awarded to members who have made significant contributions to the college or general practice development.

Benefits of membership include the monthly *British Journal of General Practice (BJGP),* discounts on RCGP publications and benefits of the local faculties. Hotel and conference accommodation is available in London.

The college also offers educational bursaries specifically for GPs in training and Education Fellowships for GPs carrying out research in GP settings.

Academic Departments of General Practice and Primary Care

Each medical school has a Department of General Practice or Primary Care that has a responsibility for undergraduate and postgraduate teaching as well as research. They may undertake research locally and nationally and in conjunction with other specialty departments.†

† See Academic posts, p. 266.

Royal Society of Medicine

Based in central London, the Royal Society of Medicine (RSM) provides a forum for education and exchange of ideas in all medical fields. It has an excellent GP section with regular academic meetings and superb library. It also has a good restaurant and inexpensive accommodation for members.

SOURCES AND FURTHER READING

1. General Medical Council website, www.gmc-uk.org
2. Department of Health website, www.doh.gov.uk
3. The National Health Service website, www.nhs.uk
4. Health of Wales Information Service website, www.wales.nhs.uk
5. Scottish Executive Health Department in Scotland website, www.show.scot.nhs.uk
6. Department of Health, Social Services and Public Safety in Northern Ireland website, www.dhsspsni.gov.uk
7. National Institute of Clinical Excellence website, www.nice.org.uk
8. Commission for Health Improvement website, www.chi.nhs.uk
9. National Patient Safety Agency website, www.npsa.org.uk

10. NHS Direct website, www.nhsdirect.nhs.uk
11. British Medical Association website, www.bma.org.uk
12. General Practitioners Committee via the BMA website, www.bma.org/gpc.nsf
13. National Association of Non-Principals website, www.nanp.org.uk
14. Joint Committee on Postgraduate Training for General Practice website, www.jcptgp.org
15. Royal College of General Practitioners website, www.rcgp.org.uk
16. Royal Society of Medicine website, www.roysocmed.ac.uk

5
The induction period and planning your year

INTRODUCTION

Your first 2 weeks in your GP registrar post should be a fully timetabled introduction to the practice and team. You should still have some protected time even if it is not your first registrar post.

To help you have a relatively clear head when you start consulting, use this time to start organizing your:

* See Chapter 6: The GP registrar contract and finances.

† See Chapter 7: Practical preparations for clinical work.

‡ See section E: The educational content of the year, Chapters 19–22.

- personal administration*
- basic equipment for consulting†
- educational plans.‡

Ensure you have access to the current editions of the essential training and reference materials for the year (*Box 5.1*). The deanery educational pack, complete with your summative assessment pack, should find its way to you automatically. You may have to track the others down yourself.

Read chapters 2–4 so you begin to understand who's who and how general practice works. Establish your basic weekly timetable with your trainer and let your practice manager know of any leave you have already organized.

Box 5.1   Essential GP registrar training and reference materials

Contract, leave and finance	*GP Registrars' Pack* from the GP Registrars' Subcommittee of the General Practitioners Committee of the BMA
Education	Deanery educational pack (and website address for updates)
Summative Assessment	Summative assessment pack (included in above) containing national summative assessment guidelines Video equipment
The MRCGP Exam	Latest regulations from the RCGP examinations department
JCPTGP Certification	*A Guide to Certification* from the JCPTGP

INTRODUCTION TO THE PRACTICE (*BOX 5.2*)

Keep a notebook (or electronic organizer) to jot down vital information, personal codes and instructions relevant to practice systems during your tour (*Box 5.3*). Collect useful phone numbers as you go.* There is a lot to take in so do not expect to remember it all.

* See Useful contacts proforma, inside back cover.

Practice staff

You should be introduced to and welcomed by all the staff. Actively introduce yourself to anyone inadvertently omitted by your trainer.

Box 5.2   Introduction to the practice

Practice tour (*see Box 5.3*)

Introduction to practice staff

Introduction to practice systems:
- computers including training, password and printers
- appointments
- results
- post and paperwork
- repeat prescriptions
- phones
- messages
- internal communications including e-mail
- on-call arrangements
- health authority claims

Sitting in with:
- trainer
- other partners
- in-house staff: practice nurse
- key members of the primary health care team (see Chapter 3)
- community services: pharmacist, podiatrist, social services, funeral directors

Reception duties:
- phones
- booking appointments
- filing

Sitting in the waiting room

Box 5.3   Practice tour

Building
- Keys for practice
- Practice alarm system (whose responsibility?)
- Locking up procedure
- Parking arrangements

Safety
- Panic alarm system
- Fire drill and escapes
- Accident book
- Sharps injury protocol

Communications
- Phone system
- Bleep system for visits and out of hours
- E-mail
- Pathology laboratory personal ID code
- Fax

Staff organization
- Staff who's who
- Partners' half-days/visiting days
- Duty doctor rota
- Protocol for leave requests

Clinical
- Tour of treatment room/clinical supplies
- Resuscitation equipment
- Access to drug cupboard and controlled drugs
- Vaccines storage

Paperwork
- In and out trays (specimens, notes and post)
- Dictaphone and tapes
- Stationery supplies and spare batteries

Refreshment
- Coffee and tearoom (kitty contributions?)
- Staff toilets
- Staff lockers

Use this time to befriend reception staff who will be extremely helpful to you later. Primary Health Care Team* members are often keen to meet you too and will want to instil in you good referral habits for your mutual benefit. Find out who works where, how to contact them and which patient groups they cover.

* See Chapter 3: Other professionals working in primary care

Making the most of sitting in

Observe actively when you sit in with partners and other staff. With the GPs compare:

- their consulting styles and speed
- the types of patients they see
- how much they prescribe
- how much they refer.

Find out their special interests both in and outside medicine. Are they hanging on for early retirement or ready to embrace yet another change in the NHS?

With non-medical colleagues, gain an insight into their qualifications, training, salary (if you dare ask), hours and general job description. Ask about the highs and lows of their jobs and how to get the best from their service.

Practice systems

Your trainer should go through all the practice systems (see *Box 5.2*) and the basic paperwork, forms and processes (including health authority claims)† you need for your daily clinical work.

†See NHS income, p.19.

The induction weeks and early tutorials should particularly focus on these; each chapter in Section D – Day-to-Day Clinical Work of the GP Registrar, could be used as a starting point. It is worth keeping sample copies of commonly used forms‡ with reminder notes of how they are used.

‡ See General practice forms, p. 271.

The importance of having water-tight practice systems is high-lighted in Chapter 23: Guidance for Good Professional Practice.

PLANNING YOUR YEAR

> **Do not let your educational needs be submerged by service interests.**

Sit down with your trainer to plan the year objectively. Individualize your requirements according to your past clinical experience and confidence. Use year planners and other useful props supplied in your deanery training pack. You should review and revise your plans at least every 3 months.

Distinguish your clinical objectives from educational ones in your plans and always keep in mind the bottom-line aims of the year:

- confidence to conduct a surgery safely and efficiently
- successful completion of summative assessment
- acquisition of your JCPTGP certificate.

These will help you to focus when your daily clinical work threatens to take over.

The clinical year

You will start with a hospital-influenced approach and be quite dependent on your trainer. As you progress, your autonomy will increase and you should ultimately be working independently in 'partnership' with your GP colleagues.

As you gain clinical experience use the categories of the summative assessment Structured Trainer's Report* to focus your professional development.

* See Structured Trainer's Report, p. 199.

By the end of the year you should be able to manage the following confidently:

- 'bread and butter' general practice medicine
- psychosocial problems
- chronic diseases and conditions
- health promotion and screening, and
- emergencies in a GP setting.

You should also have insight into:

- how general practice is run and managed as a business; and
- general practice in the wider context of the ever-changing NHS.

You do *not* need to run your own minor surgery clinic, do all your own home deliveries, become a police surgeon and manage the practice staff yet!

The educational year

See also Section E – The Educational Content of the Year.

The basic framework of your educational year will be set by the requirements of summative assessment and the MRCGP exam modules. Familiarize yourself with their current requirements in your first month* and fill in your year planner with the submission deadlines and exam dates together with dates of all regional courses. The GP press regularly publishes year planners with current summative assessment and MRCGP exam dates.

* See Chapters 20, 21 and 22.

Work out with your trainer which additional GP skills and qualifications† you can reasonably expect to acquire in the year.

† See Useful skills and qualifications, p. 190.

Try to keep your first few months clear of anything extra unless you have already applied to sit one of the diploma exams.‡ As the year goes on do not overload yourself – be selective. Your training will by no means be finished by the end of the year and there is plenty in the day-to-day work to occupy you.

‡ See Diploma exams, p. 192.

YOUR TIMETABLE

Your basic weekly timetable (*Box 5.4*) should include your visiting schedule and the duty and out-of-hours rota. If your sessions do not coincide exactly with your trainer's then establish who will be supervising you in their absence.

Antenatal, well-baby or other specialist clinics are a useful part of your training. Agree to these only when you feel sufficiently skilled and supervised.

Box 5.4   Basic GP registrar week

Full-time registrar
• six or seven clinical sessions
• tutorial
• VTS release course
• half-day off
• protected time for summative assessment obligations

Include in your own timetable practice meetings and a slot for outstanding paperwork. Make a note of local postgraduate centre and PCG/PCT meetings. Your timetable may change from week to week.

Aim to get away early on your half-day so it really is that, and not just 2 hours. You shouldn't necessarily be expected to do visits beforehand.

SOURCES AND FURTHER READING

1. Hall M., Dwyer D., Lewis T. *The GP Training Handbook*, 3rd edn. Blackwell Science, 1999.
2. BMA General Practitioners Committee. *GP Registrars' Pack*, May 2001 (guidance also available on BMA website, www.bma.org.uk).
3. JCPTGP. *A Guide to Certification*, 2001.
4. Committee of General Practice Education Directors. *Summative Assessment for General Practice Training,* August 2001 (also known as the 'Protocol'). Available at www.doctoronline.nhs.uk or in paper copy from the National Office for Summative Assessment, m.attwood@wkac.ac.uk

6
The GP registrar contract and finances

INTRODUCTION

Working conditions and salary for the GP registrar year differ from hospital training posts so get yourself organized to ensure you are properly remunerated.

One of the key features of the year is that you are supernumerary to the service requirements of the practice. As such your working arrangements should reflect your training needs and not the practice's workload.

You are employed and paid by your training practice, which is in turn reimbursed by the health authority. Your basic salary includes a car allowance and out-of-hours supplement. You are eligible for other reimbursements, including your medical protection organization subscriptions, courses and some of your home telephone bill.

Use the 2-week induction period to get your basic employment administration under way and do not hesitate to ask your trainer or practice manager for advice.

The GPC Registrars' Subcommittee produces a useful registrars' pack with the latest information. Employment advice is also available to BMA members from regional BMA offices.

YOUR CONTRACT

Your trainer should provide you with a contract of employment within 8 weeks of starting your post. At the time of writing there is no national GP registrar contract but the GPC and Committee of General Practice Education Directors are drafting a model one. The advice outlined in this chapter is based on GPC guidance for a model contract from 1999 (*Box 6.1*).

Obtain separate contracts for each GP registrar post you undertake if you are not doing a continuous 12-month stretch in the same practice, or if you are with the same trainer for two or more distinct periods.

Your trainer may also set out a specific non-compulsory educational

* See Educational contract, p. 186.

contract.*

Protecting your workload

> **You must always be supervised whenever you are on duty.**

Although you will make a significant clinical contribution to the practice you should be considered a luxury and not a workhorse! You

Box 6.1 Key inclusions of GP registrar contract

Basic stipulations
- Duration of post
- Notice on either side: usually 1 month, written.
- Salary and car allowance
- Superannuation contributions
- Obligation to have recognized medical protection organization membership

Hours
- Stipulated for:
  - work
  - tuition
  - assessment
  - VTS release course (considered part of the working week).
- Out-of-hours commitment

Leave entitlement (pro rata for part-timers)
- Annual leave: 5 weeks plus statutory and national holidays or days in lieu.
- Study leave
- Sick leave: see Red Book for payments.
- Maternity leave
- Paternity leave
- Other leave, e.g. parental leave, for GP registrar representation

Duties and responsibilities of trainer
- Ensure supervision whenever GP registrar on duty
- Install GP registrar home phone line and bedroom extension if necessary
- Cover all answering service costs
- Provide all equipment for training purposes

Duties and responsibilities of registrar
- Live at stipulated address
- Keep and maintain suitable transport
- Keep medical records
- Protect practice and patient confidentiality
- Negotiate other outside work activities, whether paid or not

may need to negotiate your workload with your trainer so you can maximize the training and educational benefits of the year. This becomes more relevant as the year progresses and your clinical workload increases. You should not:

- work more than the average full-timer at the practice or do more out-of-hours work (pro rata for part-timers)
- be involved in work that generates private income for the practice unless it is of educational value to you.*

* See Non-NHS income, p. 20 and Charging for extras, p. 159.

† See also Chapter 18: Out-of-hours work.

Out-of-hours work†

You need enough out-of-hours experience to prepare you for independent practice, but this should not mean you participate in unfair rotas. There are currently no defined national requirements for GP registrars and there are widespread variations. The GPC recommends between 1 and 10 million patient hours (a 6-hour session at a cooperative covering 100 000 patients provides 600 000 patient hours – pro rata where there is more than one doctor on duty). Recommendations may be set locally amongst trainers and the Director should be informed of the out-of-hours arrangements for their registrars.

The following points are intended to protect you from abuse:

- your trainer must be involved in providing out-of-hours care themselves (some GPs opt out of undertaking the work altogether and pay for the service)
- you should not undertake any out-of-hours duties alone for the first month, but you should use this time to accompany your trainer
- you must be supervised at all times out-of-hours by your trainer or a nominated supervisor. Although phone supervision is acceptable, the supervising doctor must be able to join you if you request it
- you should not undertake any work for which you feel ill-equipped
- you are not allowed to receive additional payment for out-of-hours work or be employed by a cooperative (see 'Your basic salary' below)
- you should not be expected to do any night work the day before the VTS release course, and should always have time off in the practice in the day following any night work you do.

Leave entitlements

Study leave

JCPTGP guidance states that GP registrars should have a minimum of 30 days a year for the VTS release course and study leave. There is no maximum study leave allowance stipulated. Your total study leave will depend on your educational needs, balanced with the needs of your practice that may take precedence. Negotiate your requirements with your trainer.

Additional protected time may be negotiated for work relating to summative assessment.

Sick leave

If you are ill phone your trainer and/or practice manager on the first day of illness. Give them a realistic idea of how long you will need to be off to allow the practice manager to make appropriate arrangements, cancel your surgeries and ensure you are fully productive when you return to work. You should forewarn them, particularly if you expect to be off for a week or more.

Provided you were employed when you first became ill you are entitled to sick pay as stipulated in the Red Book. You will not be covered for any time you remain ill after your GP registrar contract expires if you have no other employment set up. Your practice manager will need a medical certificate from your own GP for illness longer than 7 days.*

* See Sickness certificates, p. 146.

Maternity leave

Rights to maternity leave are granted by your practice rather than the NHS.

Discuss with your trainer, practice manager and the BMA how to maximize your paid leave entitlements. Generally speaking you need to have at least 12 months' continuous NHS service (in hospital or as a GP registrar) to qualify. Rates are quoted in the back of *Medeconomics*. You may be entitled to Statutory Maternity Pay (SMP) but you will need to check this. Your practice manager will need a MATB1 certificate from you from week 20.†

† See Maternity certificates, p. 151.

Paternity leave

As there is no current statutory right to paternity leave this is at the discretion of the practice. Any leave granted is likely to be unpaid and probably up to a maximum of 2 weeks, as in hospital service.

Parental leave

For each child born or adopted after 15th December 1999, up to 13 weeks of unpaid leave are allowable. These must be taken in periods of not less than a week and before the child's fifth birthday, or fifth anniversary of adoption.

As this statutory entitlement depends on 12 months' continuous service it doesn't automatically apply to GP registrars so you may need to incorporate it into your contract if relevant.

Other leave

* See GP political, p. 41. GP registrars representing their grade on recognized bodies* are entitled to additional leave for this with the agreement of their trainer.

Discuss compassionate leave with your trainer should the need arise.

Your training period must be extended accordingly for any lengthy unpaid leave you take.

Other contractual stipulations

Your contract should state that you have your own suitable transport, not necessarily a car, and keep it serviced. Relevant allowances are covered below.

The practice should provide all equipment and clinical supplies for your day-to-day work and summative assessment, but you should buy † See Your medical bag, p. 64. core equipment for your medical bag.† Keep any borrowed equipment in good condition and return or replace it at the end of the year.

Difficulties arising with your contract

If you feel your trainer or practice is in breach of your contract or problems arise during the year, approach your trainer in the first ‡ See also Making the most of your trainer, p. 186. instance.‡ If you feel it would be impossible to do so then consider discussing it with your VTS course organizer or Director. Serious employment issues may be taken up with an arbitrator via the BMA for members.

GP REGISTRAR FINANCES

> **Keep receipts for all medical and course-related expenses.**

Your basic salary

Your basic starting salary depends on your previous NHS post and your incremental date will continue from your hospital post. Exceptions exist where your previous post was a locum, overseas or in the armed forces.

GP registrar salaries are agreed nationally and pay scales are set out in the Department of Health statement *Directions to Health Authorities Concerning GP Registrars* (which also outlines the other reimbursements due). They can also be found in the GPC GP registrars' pack and at the back of *Medeconomics*.

Your salary automatically includes an out-of-hours supplement, calculated at a percentage of the basic salary.

National Insurance and superannuation contributions

Your national insurance and superannuation contributions should be deducted from your gross salary at source. Check this is the case on your first pay slip and discuss with your practice manager if is not. The practice pays the employer's share, which is refunded by the health authority.

Getting paid

Your practice manager should let you know what documentation is needed to confirm your previous post and salary scale. You will need to complete some paperwork for the health authority and you may need your passport or birth certificate to confirm your age for pension purposes. You will also need your P45 and emergency tax will be deducted from your pay until this is received.

You should be paid by direct transfer to your bank in arrears at the end of each completed month, but you may be paid by cheque for your first month while the practice and health authority get themselves organized.

Allowances and reimbursements (Box 6.2)

Your salary includes a car allowance, with proportional payments for flexible trainees, and for motorcycles and mopeds (see Tax return below), except for those on paid maternity leave.

London weighting is included for practices in London and a defined fringe area.

You may be eligible for other reimbursements, which should be claimed from your deanery or the health authority, through your practice manager. Keep all receipts.

Medical protection organization subscriptions

You are obliged to have medical protection cover as a GP registrar and are entitled to reimbursement for the amount of the GP registrar rate

Box 6.2   GP registrar allowances and reimbursements

Allowances
- London weighting where applicable
- Car allowance to cover petrol, expenses, servicing (33% for motorcycles >50 cc; 20% for mopeds or motorcycles ≤50 cc)

Reimbursements
- Course fees for Section 63-approved courses
- Removal and associated relocation expenses
- Travel and subsistence for:
  - searching for accommodation
  - attending interview for GP registrar post
  - sitting a postgraduate qualification (not exam fees)
  - attending an approved study leave course.
- Medical protection organization subscription
- Phone:
  - cost of installing a bedroom phone extension (if essential for your work)
  - cost of rental charge for your home phone if you pay it
  - mobile phone costs are not reimbursable.

subscription less the basic subscription. Your practice manager will need your certificate to organize reimbursement, which can be paid monthly, or in one lump sum, depending on how you pay your subscription.

Additional fees

Find out from the practice manager or your trainer if you are allowed to keep any fees generated by private work you do for the practice such as completion of cremation forms, Medical Attendant's Reports or solicitor's reports.* Practices may pool all such income or direct it to the doctor who undertook the work. Keep a record of any fees you receive for tax purposes.

* See Charging for extras, p. 159.

Study leave funding: Section 63

Funding for courses for GP training is available under Section 63 (of the Health Services and Public Health Act 1968) through Directors. There is an annual allocation for each GP in training whether in hospital or GP registrar post which varies from region to region. Only 'Section 63 approved' course fees can be reimbursed but most core courses suggested for vocational training should be.[†]

† See Chapter 19: Educational aspects of the year.

Claiming course fee reimbursement

Apply to your deanery office for funding approval if possible at least 6 weeks before the start of the course. Ideally await approval before booking otherwise reimbursement may not be forthcoming.

You will be sent a claim form to be completed after the course that should be submitted with a certificate of attendance, usually distributed at the end of the course. Claims for travel and subsistence expenses (for meals and overnight accommodation) associated with the course should also be submitted to the Director, together with receipts, as soon as possible after the course.

Examination fees

Although reimbursement may be available for travelling and subsistence involved in sitting an exam for a postgraduate qualification, the examination fee itself is not reimbursable.

Tax return

If you have to complete a tax return, consider employing an accountant with an interest in general practice to maximize your allowances (*Box 6.3*).

Box 6.3   General tax-allowable medical expenses

Consult your accountant for your personal allowances

Professional fees

- GMC annual retention fee
- BMA membership
- Royal colleges annual membership fee
- Medical protection organization subscriptions

Medical equipment (including spares and replaceable parts)
Business mileage
Business phone costs

Reproduced from the BMA Website, Tax guidance.

Books, journals, examination and course fees are generally not tax-allowable, but you should be reimbursed for most of the courses you attend during this year anyway.

If your car allowance is taxed at source you may be able to offset this with business mileage costs. These include travel from your home to emergency visits and day-time visits from the surgery, but exclude travel from home to your place of work. Keep a record in a notebook in your car.

SOURCES AND FURTHER READING

1. BMA General Practitioners Committee. *Guidance for GP Registrars*, November 1999.
2. BMA General Practitioners Committee. *GP Registrars' Pack*, May 2001 (available on BMA website at www.bma.org.uk).
3. Department of Health. *Directions for Health Authorities concerning GP Registrars*, April 2001.
4. Tax guidance from the BMA website, www.bma.org.uk

7
Practical preparations for clinical work

INTRODUCTION

You will need to buy a medical bag and some essential equipment for yourself, but your practice should provide the clinical supplies and paperwork for your everyday work together with drugs for your bag. Borrow from the practice before you buy anything. The GP newspapers often have a clinical equipment mail order section, which may be cheaper than specialist medical shops. Keep all your receipts for tax purposes.

The recommendations here are based on personal use and what our local cooperatives use. They are intended as prompts (for you, your trainer and your practice manager) and not as prescriptive lists. Discuss your personal requirements with your trainer.

The order within the lists (except those for drugs) relates roughly to how frequently you will use the supplies. Additional preparations for visiting are covered in Chapter 17: Home Visits.

YOUR MEDICAL BAG

This must be lockable and ideally quite light. Anything advertised as a medical bag may be expensive and offer no advantages over a cheaper alternative such as a briefcase, toolbox or vanity case.

Insure your bag and its contents on your household insurance. If you have to leave it in your car make sure both the bag, and the car, are locked.

You are responsible for your own bag so restock it regularly.

Equipment and clinical supplies

Unless you have a double set of everything, your main equipment will be used both in surgery and on visits. What you need (*Box 7.1*) will depend on where you practise, how much on-call you do and how organized you like to be. Those working in remoter areas may need more emergency equipment, such as a nebulizer, i.v. fluids, Venflons and a defibrillator, than their town counterparts.

Use the following tips when you first stock your bag:

- keep related clinical supplies together in labelled plastic bags or boxes
- carry a limited selection of dressings and bandages for first-aid purposes only and leave more complicated dressings to the district nurses

Box 7.1   Your medical bag

Equipment
- Stethoscope
- Portable sphygmomanometer
- Ophthalmoscope/auriscope
- Thermometer (ideally aural infra-red)
- Peak flow meter, mouthpieces and PEFR calculator
- Patella hammer
- Tape measure (for DVTs/obstetrics)
- Laerdal pocket mask and oropharyngeal airway
- Scissors

Clinical supplies
- Drugs (*see Boxes 7.2 and 7.3*)
- Spare medicine bottles or envelopes to dispense medicines
- Tongue depressors
- Urine pots
- Urinalysis sticks
- Gloves
- KY jelly
- Lancets and BM stix or glucometer
- Venesection equipment:
    - needles, butterflies, syringes and blood bottles
    - cotton wool and plasters
    - specimens bags.
- Tourniquet
- Disinfecting swabs (for cleaning skin and ear pieces)
- Venflons
- Pregnancy test kit and gestation calculator
- Dressing pack and some simple dressings and tape
- Fluorescein strips

General
- Mini sharps box
- Rubbish receptacle

Paperwork
- Folder/wallet with pockets for selection of paperwork, headed paper, envelopes
- List of practice and hospital phone numbers*
- Reference charts of emergency drug doses and anything else you may not remember

* See Useful contacts proforma, inside back cover.

Books
- *British National Formulary (BNF)*
- Notebook for patient details, interesting cases, claims for night visits and temporary residents
- Local A–Z or map

- you will not necessarily need Venflons too as i.v. drugs can be given via a butterfly or syringe
- a paediatric stethoscope is not essential
- aural thermometers are excellent for quick temperatures
- carry 'Multistix' if possible; although expensive, they are useful for assessing ketones and UTIs. Make sure the sticks in the bottle match the guide and have not been topped up from another bottle
- your practice will usually order in ear-pieces, and provide batteries for equipment.

* See also Chapter 10: Prescribing and Using drugs out of hours, p. 181.

Drugs for your bag* (Boxes 7.2 and 7.3)

> **Ensure drugs are in date when you check your medical bag.**

† See Sources and further reading.

There is an essential minimum you must carry. Marked '**' in *Box 7.2*, these are potentially life-saving treatments for myocardial infarction, cardiac arrest, asthma, anaphylaxis, hypoglycaemia, meningococcal infection or psychosis. *The Drug and Therapeutics Bulletin* has published a useful guide to appropriate drugs (and doses) to carry for use in emergencies.† Discuss which other drugs to carry with your trainer.

Box 7.2 Emergency drugs

Remember vials of water for injection

Condition	Suggested quantity to carry (for doses see *BNF*)
Anaphylaxis	• Adrenaline (Epinephrine)** 1 ml 1 in 1000 (=1 mg/ml) vials × 2
	• Chlorphenamine (Chlorpheniramine)** 1 ml (10 mg/ml) injection × 1
	• Hydrocortisone** powder (as succinate) 100 mg × 2 with 2 × 2 ml water for reconstitution. Also for asthma and hypoadrenalism
Asthma	• Salbutamol nebules 2.5 ml (1 mg/ml) × 2 *or* Terbutaline nebules 2 ml (2.5 mg/ml) × 2
	• Salbutamol metered dose inhaler × 1 *or* Terbutaline MDI × 1
	• Prednisolone** 5 mg soluble tablets × 8

	• Hydrocortisone i.v., see above
	• Ipratropium nebules 1 ml (250 μg/ml) × 2
	• Aminophylline i.v. solution 10 ml (25 mg/ml) × 2
Cardiac:	
Suspected MI	• Aspirin** tablets (soluble or chewable) 300 mg × 10
	• GTN spray × 1
	• Diamorphine** vial dry powder for reconstitution 5 mg × 2
	• Metoclopramide 2 ml (5 mg/ml) vial × 1
	• Cyclizine 1 ml (50 mg/ml) vial × 1
Acute LVF	• Furosemide (Frusemide)** 5 ml (10 mg/ml) vial × 1
	• Diamorzphine as above
Bradycardia	• Atropine** 1 ml vial (600 μg/ml) × 1
Diabetic hypoglycaemia	• Glucose tablets or 3 sugar lumps (= 10 g) *or*
	• Hypostop gel 23 g oral ampoule × 1
	• Glucagon** 1 mg/ml injection × 1
	• Glucose i.v. solution 50 ml of 20%
Epileptic fit or febrile convulsion	• Rectal Diazepam** 1.25 ml (2 mg/ml) × 1 (= 2.5 mg) *and* 2.5 ml (2 mg/ml) × 2 (= 10 mg total) *or*
	• Diazepam emulsion 2 ml (5 mg/ml) vial × 1 Also for psychotic agitation
Meningococcal disease	• Benzylpenicillin** dry powder vials for reconstitution 2 × 600 mg ('GP pack')
	• For confirmed penicillin allergy: Cefotaxime** powder for reconstitution 1 g vial × 1 *or* Chloramphenicol powder for reconstitution 1 g vial × 1
Psychiatric – agitated psychotic	• Chlorpromazine** 1 ml (25 mg/ml) vial × 2 *or*
	• Haloperidol 1 ml (5 mg/ml) vial × 2 (can also be used for vomiting)
Antidotes	• Flumazenil 5 ml (100 μg/ml) vial × 1
	• Naloxone 1 ml (400 μg/ml) vial × 2
	• Procyclidine 2 ml (5 mg/ml) vial × 2
Analgesia	• Diamorphine as above
	• Tramadol 2 ml (50 mg/ml) vial × 1
	• Diclofenac 3 ml (25 mg/ml) vial × 1

"Drugs for the Doctor's Bag Revisited" – *Drug and Therapeutics Bulletin*, (Vol. 38, No. 9, September 2000) reproduced with kind permission by Consumers' Association, 2 Marylebone Road, London, NW1 4DF.

* See Controlled drugs,
p. 106.

Carry the emergency drugs grouped by condition and keep the vials in a plastic box cushioned with foam, together with water for injection.

Familiarize yourself with the regulations on the carriage and storage of controlled drugs (CDs).* Doctors have been prosecuted for contravening these regulations so you *must* observe them.

Box 7.3   Oral preparations for your medical bag

Drug group	Suggested quantity to carry (for doses see *BNF*)
Analgesics/ antipyretics	• Paracetamol soluble tablets 500 mg × 10 • Paracetamol sugar-free (SF) solution 120 mg/5 ml × 100 ml • Ibuprofen 200 mg tablets × 10 • Ibuprofen SF solution 100 mg/5 ml × 100 ml • Diclofenac 50 mg tablets × 10 • Dihydrocodeine 30 mg tablets × 10
Antibiotics	• Amoxicillin 250 mg tablets × 12 • Amoxicillin SF powder 125 mg/5 ml (reconstituted 1 bottle = 100 ml) • Erythromycin 250 mg tablets × 12 • Erythromycin SF powder 125 mg/5 ml (reconstituted = 140 ml) • Trimethoprim 200 mg tablets × 8 • Trimethoprim SF suspension 50 mg/5 ml × 100 ml • Flucloxacillin 250 mg tablets × 12 • Flucloxacillin SF powder 125 mg/5 ml (reconstituted = 100 ml)
Anti-emetic	• Prochlorperazine buccal tablets 3 mg × 12
Antacid	• Packet of Gaviscon or magnesium trisilicate tablets • Cimetidine 200 mg × 10
Antihistamine	• Chlorphenamine 4 mg tablets × 10
Oral rehydration solution sachets	• Any make × 6

"Drugs for the Doctor's Bag Revisited" – *Drug and Therapeutics Bulletin*, (Vol. 38, No. 9, September, 2000) reproduced with kind permission by Consumers' Association, 2 Marylebone Road, London, NW1 4DF.

Carry a bottle of amoxicillin and erythromycin. Antibiotic starter packs supplied by drug reps are rarely generic or first-line recommendations.

Ordering drug supplies

Your drugs may come from practice stocks or be ordered in specially. Find out whose job this is and present them with a list of what you need. Alternatively you may need to write out a private prescription* for the local pharmacist.

* See Private prescriptions, p. 109.

Practice (and personal) drug stocks are initially paid for by the practice or individual GP. They can be replenished, from a local pharmacy, by writing an NHS prescription in the patient's name whenever you dispense any drug or dressing from your bag or from the surgery. Do so even if you dispense only two paracetamol tablets.

Keep limited supplies of drugs. You may not use them frequently (and they will just go out of date) and most patients will have access to a pharmacy within 24–48 hours of a visit anyway. Cooperatives may provide drugs for use in their sessions.

Dispensing drugs from your bag

Transfer drugs from your supplies into spare medicine bottles or an envelope you can seal. Label the container clearly with the patient's name, date, full drug and dose details and the number of tablets supplied. Remind the patient to store drugs safely, particularly if you dispense them into envelopes.

Document in the medical records the batch number, expiry date and, if appropriate, manufacturer of any drugs you actually administer yourself, particularly i.v. or vaccinations.†

† See Drug and product liability, p. 111.

YOUR CONSULTING ROOM

Ideally you should have your own consulting room, which should be cleared of all your predecessor's debris and restocked for your arrival (*Box 7.4*). If you have to share a room, or move between rooms, keep your personal affairs and notes separate and clearly identifiable as yours (use plastic baskets).

Make your room comfortable both for you and your patients. Organize it and add personal touches in your induction period (*Box 7.5*). Find out who is responsible for restocking it and make sure you know where supplies are kept for the times (usually out-of-hours) when they are not around.

Keep in mind health and safety issues in the layout of your room. All sharps bins and dangerous equipment should be out of children's reach and prescription and medical certificate pads kept out of sight. Measures to protect yourself from the occasional potentially violent interaction are covered in Chapter 8: Ground Rules Before You Start Consulting.

A cluttered desk can easily add to your sense of chaos so try to keep your desktop and drawers tidy. The stationery you will need (*Box 7.6*) will depend on the type of notes used (Lloyd George, A4) and the degree of computerization of the practice. Paper-lean practices still use plenty of paper.

Box 7.4   Clinical equipment for the consulting room

As for your medical bag (*Box 7.1*) plus

Equipment
- Weighing scales
- Height meter
- Snellen chart (and mark the distance from which the patient should read it)

Clinical supplies
- Disposable gloves
- Microbiology, chlamydia swabs
- Gynaecology examination equipment: specula, spatula, cytobrush, slides, fixative, pencil, slide carriers
- Box of tissues
- Plastic specimen bags
- Sharps bin

Access to
- Drug cupboard
- Vaccines fridge
- Anaphylaxis kit
- Oxygen
- Nebulizer and nebules
- Placebo inhalers and spacer device for demonstration
- Foetal heart monitor and water-soluble jelly (KY works as well)
- Proctoscope
- Minor surgery equipment
- Pregnancy test kits
- Family planning kit, including demonstration models
- Mycology sample kits
- Eye examination equipment: fluorescein, dilating drops, saline, blue light
- Ear syringing kit
- Spare batteries
- Other equipment (e.g. ECG machine, spirometer, electrocautery, etc.)

Box 7.5　Personal organization for your room

General
- Door nameplate
- Personalized practice stamp
- Clock
- Pinboard/whiteboard and marker
- Calendar/year planner

Desk
- Pots for pencils, tongue depressors
- Hole punch, stapler, sticky tape and dispenser
- Paperclips, rubber bands, treasury tags, drawing pins

Filing
- Baskets for patients' notes for 'action'
- In-tray or magazine files for accumulated paperwork
- Card index box
- Filing cabinet or drawer
- Bookshelf

Other
- Personalizing effects (photos, pictures, plants, your own mug, radio, aromatherapy)
- Basket of toys (washable and disinfectable – not soft toys)
- Reward stickers for brave children
- Access to video equipment

Keep your notebook of useful information and patient queries to hand when you are consulting.

REFERENCE MATERIAL*

* See also Chapter 15: Paperwork, Drug information sources, p. 112 and Databases, p. 122.

You will need clinical reference material, information for patient referrals and patient information leaflets (*Box 7.7*) for your day-to-day work, much of which may be on the practice computer. Your trainer and other practice staff, particularly the secretary, will also be helpful. Build up your own collection and keep it filed for easy access during surgery.

Discuss in a tutorial how best to deal with the constant stream of material received by post.

Box 7.6   Everyday stationery

- Lloyd George continuation cards (FP7 and 8: male = red, female = blue) or A4 continuation sheets
- Surgery headed notepaper, envelopes and compliments slips.
- Prescription forms FP10 and FP10 comp
- Request forms for pathology, radiology and local services.
- Medical certificates: Meds 3, 4, 5, DS1500
- Maternity claims paperwork (GMS3 and FW8 prescription exemption application)
- Termination forms (HSΛ1 form)
- Patient information leaflets
- Practice leaflets
- 'Post-it' notes, scrap paper, carbon paper (to duplicate hand-written letters)

Access to
- Death certificates and cremation forms
- Mental health section papers
- Referral proformas for local services
- Application for prescription exemption (FP92A)
- Medical summary card/vaccination summary
- GMS 1–4 forms (for health authority claims if not computer-linked)

Box 7.7   Suggested reference material for everyday use

Clinical
- Pregnancy gestation calculator
- Peak flow prediction calculator
- Height and weight conversion chart (imperial to metric)
- Body mass index (BMI) calculator
- Coronary heart disease risk prediction charts
- Children's growth charts
- Clinical guidelines (national and local)
- Local prescribing incentive scheme guidelines
- Practice clinical protocols, e.g. prescribing

Administrative
- Internal phone extensions
- Local hospitals directory
- Private consultants list

Books
Official publications (see Recommended Reading)
- The *BNF* (rather than *MIMS*)
- *Clinical Evidence*
- Practice or local formulary (if available)
- Guide to 'over-the-counter' (OTC) drugs
- *Immunisation Against Infectious Disease* ('The Green book')
- *Department of Health Guide to Travel Vaccinations* ('The Yellow book')
- Fitness to drive *'At a Glance'* guide

Clinical reference texts
- A clinical GP reference
- *Oxford Handbooks of Clinical Medicine and Specialties*
- *Oxford Handbook of Patients' Welfare*
- A family planning reference book
- A dermatology atlas
- ENT, ophthalmology, musculoskeletal, etc., reference

SOURCES AND FURTHER READING

1. Drugs for the Doctor's Bag Revisited, including insert: 'Parenteral Doses of Drugs for Medical Emergencies', *Drug and Therapeutics Bulletin* **38** (9), 2000.
2. Current *BNF*.
   See Recommended Reading for reference texts.

8
Ground rules before you start consulting

INTRODUCTION

Here we suggest a few basic rules that will help to ground you during the inevitable times when you feel out of your depth. You may need to remind yourself and even your trainer, from time to time, of these basic tenets.

SUPERVISION

* See Protecting your workload, p. 54.

Your trainer has a responsibility for your actions in all aspects of your work so they must be confident that you are clinically competent and ensure adequate supervision whenever you are on duty.* You retain clinical responsibility for your work so you need adequate medical protection organization cover.

In your trainer's absence there must be another nominated partner, not necessarily a trainer, to take on this supervisory role. Identify who this is and do not hesitate to use them.

ASKING FOR HELP

It is a rare luxury in medical training to have your own individual tutor and mentor so make good use of them. Use every opportunity to ask questions and ask for their help on clinical, administrative and service-related issues, but be sensitive to their workload and time pressures.

This is also the time to fill many of the black holes in your clinical knowledge base. Everyone has them, including your trainer. Do not be embarrassed by your ignorance of what you might perceive to be trivial queries ('What *are* chilblains'?). You will gain respect by asking and the worst that can happen is that you will have to look it up yourself or even present a practice meeting on the subject!

Urgent queries

You may often need help or advice mid-surgery, particularly early in the year. If it cannot wait until after surgery then do not hesitate to ask your trainer or another partner. It is not unusual for registrars to hover outside their trainer's door hoping to pounce between patients.

Avoid frustrating waits for you and your patient by prioritizing your need for help according to the situation. Spend a couple of minutes clarifying exactly what it is you want before you ask. If you need your trainer's second opinion then say so straightaway: 'Could you come and see this 2-year-old with an unusual facial rash?' Ask your trainer if they are happy to be phoned mid-surgery for simple queries.

Remember that your trainer, or supervising partner, may be under some pressure themselves (in the middle of a difficult consultation or racing out to do a mental health section), so do not take it personally if you get short shrift. You will simply have to wait or ask someone else; the practice as a whole should support your training needs.

Other queries

These are things that can wait until after surgery, the next tutorial, your paperwork catch-up slot or even the VTS meeting. Keep your notebook on your desk to keep track of queries. Aim to look up things at home as soon as possible; there will be more queries tomorrow.

You will need to ask for advice from your hospital colleagues, including specialist registrars, pathology, radiology and pharmacy colleagues. They are usually extremely obliging. Always present your query or case clearly.

MANAGING YOUR WORKLOAD

Your initial workload will be less onerous than a full-time partner's but as the year progresses you will probably find that there is too much expected in the time available. Aside from surgeries, the work arising from the constant stream of unplanned 'extras' can be extremely time-consuming.*

There is usually a continual demand from staff and patients for small tasks that will 'only take 2 minutes' but invariably take longer. Unless there is an obvious medical emergency, avoid reacting 'stat' to each episode. Instead, prioritize and agree pleasantly to do the task when it suits you. If you do agree there and then, such as when a receptionist begs for a prescription for a waiting patient, ensure you give it your full clinical attention and do not allow yourself to be rushed. Sometimes it will be appropriate to refuse and ask that someone else does it instead.

* See Chapter 16: Extras in the working day.

Developing your boundaries

Do not allow yourself to be put upon, which is always a danger as the new person in the practice, since you are likely to want to be obliging. GPs simply cannot be everything to everyone so you will need to develop boundaries as to what you are prepared, and able, to do for your patients, staff and colleagues. These boundaries will inevitably change with time and experience. Good boundary keeping may explain why some of your colleagues appear to make themselves unavailable at times. The most conscientious doctors may have difficulty setting boundaries and so be prone to burnout.

LOOKING AFTER YOURSELF

General practice can be a very busy and stressful job, wherever it is practised. Your tutorials, VTS group and texts on the consultation will cover the issues of 'housekeeping' and stress management but here are a few tips to keep you mentally well and full of enthusiasm for the job in years to come. They may take some practice to achieve:

* learn to say *no* on occasion
* delegate where appropriate so long as you are confident that whoever you ask is up to the task
* give yourself reasonable planning time before launching into any task
* make time for lunch, even if it is in your car, and make meal breaks a priority when on call
* do not go more than 3 months without a proper break (holiday or study leave); ensure you really have a break and book the next one as soon as you are back
* let your trainer know if you are having personal problems, or are overwhelmed by study demands; arrangements can be made to lighten your workload
* do not let things fester – if someone's behaviour or attitude is annoying you, address the problem and confront them calmly; clear the air and move on
* learn to recognize when you are getting stressed or overtired and look after yourself – get some sleep, eat well, cancel non-essential work or social arrangements and do not agree to new tasks or projects until you are back on form.

When the going gets tough have a few stress-busting techniques up your sleeve (*Box 8.1*) which you can also recommend to your patients. Remember that prevention is always better than crisis management.

SAFETY MATTERS

There are, albeit very rare, clinical situations in which you might find yourself physically threatened. These are often unpredictable and may arise from mental illness, drug or alcohol misuse, physical illness (e.g. hypoglycaemia or head injury) or simple frustration with 'the system'. Hopefully there will be increasing awareness of the unacceptability of aggression and violence against NHS staff through the efforts of the government's NHS Zero Tolerance Zone Campaign, launched in 1999.

Box 8.1   Stress management strategies

After acutely stressful situations
- Lock your consulting room door and turn off the phone ringer
- Lie on the floor, or your examination couch
- Breathe deeply or try in one nostril, out the other
- Try muscle tensing-relaxing exercises – lying down starting with your feet, tense all foot muscles for a count of five then release for five, then tense feet and calf muscles, and relax, then feet, calf and thigh and so on until you reach the scalp and face. Concentrating on this physical activity will at least take your mind off the acute problem
- Use a squeezy stress ball
- Leave your room and put the kettle on, go to the toilet, or go for a walk around the block

Prevention
- Have a confidante, medical or otherwise, to let off steam to
- Have a laugh with your friends or partner
- Take regular physical exercise
- Have a massage
- Keep protected time for leisure activities and non-medical pastimes
- Avoid reliance on alcohol, nicotine or mind-altering substances (including television)

Prevention

You should always be open to the possibility of violence, particularly in inner-city practices. Your practice should have some basic policies for reducing the likelihood of such incidents. Ideally an identified GP should work with the practice manager and arrange regular drills in using the panic button system and meetings to discuss and learn from difficult incidents.

Ideally health authorities should provide secure facilities with surveillance equipment for consultations with patients who are known to be violent. Such facilities may be in a police station, A&E or a nominated surgery. Find out if such a facility exists locally. This should protect the GP and break the cycle of removing violent patients from a GP's list only to have them re-register elsewhere and be removed again.

The notes of previously violent patients should be marked, and specific precautions taken in the consultation. There are also general measures you can take to protect yourself (*Box 8.2*).*

* See also Visiting: safety precautions. Box 17.1, p. 170; Defusing a potentially violent situation, p. 90 and Debriefing after a difficult consultation, p. 91.

Box 8.2   Your personal safety in the consultation

- Know the panic button system, in particular:
  - location of buttons in main areas of surgery
  - how it sounds so you can respond yourself.
- Do a basic self-defence course (consider arranging a VTS session with a skilled instructor)
- Avoid consulting alone in the surgery building
- Arrange your room so your chair is nearer the exit than the patient's
- Do not go alone on a visit to a threatening patient
- Reduce throttling aids: avoid draping your stethoscope around your neck; men should consider clip-on ties
- Keep potentially dangerous instruments out of sight (scissors, scalpels, corrosive fluids)

SOURCES AND FURTHER READING

1. Schroeder, K. *Top Tips for GPs – A Beginner's Guide to General Practice.* Radcliffe Medical Press, 2000.
2. NHS Zero Tolerance Zone Campaign, www.nhs.uk/zerotolerance
3. Macdonald, R. *Violence Against NHS Staff. BMJ* (Career Focus) **322:** S2–7289, 2001.

9

The GP registrar consultation: survival tips

INTRODUCTION

There is no right or wrong way to consult, nor is there a perfect consultation. You will develop your own individual style with experience and this will evolve throughout your working life.

This chapter highlights some of the issues we found problematic, particularly early in the year. Your own experience, input from your trainer and reviews of your videos will fill in some of the gaps. Read the classic consultations texts* although you may find them a little overwhelming at the outset. When you can run your surgeries safely and comfortably use these texts to refine your consultation skills.

Always keep in mind the ground rules† and the basic aims of the year:

* See Sources and further reading.

† See Chapter 8.

- confidence to conduct a surgery safely and efficiently
- successful completion of summative assessment
- acquisition of your JCPTGP certificate.

STARTING OFF

Fundamental features of general practice consultations are:

- seeing pathology at an early, often unclear, stage and developing over time
- distinguishing the serious problems from the mundane
- dealing with uncertainty.

The transition to GP consulting

Presentations in general practice are often less well defined than in secondary care, so a different approach is needed, the main differences being:

- Full clerkings are rarely required (as the medical record should already hold a summary of the medical history), although you will hang on to these initially and be given more consulting time to account for this
- Relatively few presentations lend themselves to a clear diagnosis
- Patients often present with several problems at once
- Most presentations do not need sorting out immediately (aside from the few medical emergencies), despite the anxiety generated by worried patients and staff. You rarely need to rush out on a visit and you should resist being pressured into prompt action by socially inconvenienced patients

- Test results, and patients, take a relatively long time to come back. Whilst there is no consultant ward round to gear up for (you are now the consultant!), there is always the potential to lose patients to follow-up. Learn to share responsibility with them for follow-up of their medical problems and results. You cannot keep track of every patient in the way you are expected to as a house officer, but you should keep a note of those causing you concern
- Each consultation need not end with a prescription, investigation or referral. Simple reassurance and masterly inactivity may be entirely appropriate, but may feel rather unsettling at first.

Your early surgeries and getting up to speed

Your first solo surgeries should be very light to allow for the fact you are still in hospital clerking mode and unfamiliar with the patient, computer and general practice medicine. Progress to shorter appointment times as your confidence increases. By the end of the year you should be able to manage a surgery load similar to your trainer, including added urgent cases. Work up to this by about month four but resist pressure to do so until you are ready.

You will run late – almost all GPs do and you will get quicker with experience. Doctors are naturally fast or slow consulters and trying to change from one type to the other can be stressful and may be counterproductive. However, if running late is a persistent problem then discuss it with your trainer. You may need to make some adjustments to your approach, what you are trying to achieve in the consultation and how you organize yourself.

Do not be surprised if you feel totally exhausted in your first few weeks, although you should be working fewer hours than in your hospital jobs. This is the result of a steep learning curve, intense patient contact and the emotionally draining content of some consultations. You are also working in relative isolation and have greater clinical responsibility. However, if you were previously a medical specialist registrar you may find it all quite easy compared to outpatients.

YOUR CASE MIX

Although you will not have your own registered patients you will acquire some regulars throughout the year. Inevitably many of the cases you see will be one-off, straightforward acute medical problems. Your trainer should review your case mix with you from time to time to ensure you have a representative selection, including patients with chronic diseases, on-going psychosocial problems and someone requiring terminal care.

THE CONSULTATION ITSELF

The main practical components of the consultation (completing the medical record, prescribing, certificates, investigations and referrals) are all dealt with individually in subsequent chapters.

Conducting the consultation

* See Your consulting room, p. 69.

Your room should be welcoming and comfortable for patients.* Glance through the medical record before calling in your patient, even if you know them well, to ensure you have both the correct records to hand and the computer page visible. Most GPs call in patients directly from the waiting room. A buzzer system is quicker but less personal.

Start the consultation with a non-directive opener such as 'What can I do for you?' Do not assume you know the reason for their attendance even if you invited the patient back for review, as they may have several other issues to discuss.

Give them some uninterrupted time to tell you their reason/s for coming. After a few minutes start to explore their presenting complaint by asking direct questions.

Try to maintain eye contact and avoid excessive bonding with the computer, notes or the clock.

If it transpires that there are several problems, ask the patient to prioritize them and make it clear you will limit the consultation to what can be covered reasonably in the time available. Limit them to urgent problems only in an urgent appointment and invite them back for a further appointment, particularly if a detailed examination or a procedure is required.

When an examination is necessary ask the patient to undress only as much as is needed. Ideally you should offer a chaperone for all intimate examinations, even if you are the same gender.

Terminating the consultation can be an art in itself. Use the psychotherapist's favourite phrase, 'I'm afraid that is all we have time for today', and walk them to the door if necessary. Most patients are very sensitive to the time limits of general practice.

Follow-up and 'safety netting'

As a registrar you will ask many of your patients back for follow-up. This is partly for review following investigations or new medication, but also to reassure yourself that you are not missing something. In this way you can also observe the natural history of many self-limiting conditions.

If you are not arranging a follow-up appointment give your patient a clear invitation to return should their symptoms change or deteriorate.

Give specific guidance such as 'come back if the fever is not settling within 3 days' or 'if the breathing worsens so that the baby cannot feed easily' and document your advice clearly (TCB = to come back). You may agree on a time for a telephone review rather than a face-to-face consultation.

Some consultations will inevitably leave you feeling anxious or uncertain about your management. Discuss them with your trainer and even phone the patient later to check on progress, or inform them of revised management. They are usually very grateful for your conscientious attention. If you sense you will be left with some anxiety about a patient, particularly those with acute presentations, then trust your gut instinct and arrange a prompt review or refer them.

As you progress through the year aim to bring fewer patients back for follow-up to free up appointments.

Only through the experience of many patient contacts can you begin to achieve a balance between:

- your own learning needs in seeing the resolution or progression of conditions; and
- handing back responsibility to the patient to return appropriately.

THE CLINICAL CONTENT OF THE CONSULTATION

Broadly speaking GP clinical issues fall into the following categories:

- 'bread and butter' medicine
- psychosocial problems
- chronic diseases
- health promotion
- emergencies in general practice.

You should be well equipped from your hospital experience to deal with presentations with a clear history and obvious pathology that require referral. Deciding the priority of the referral and the extent to which you should investigate in general practice may present problems at first, so discuss queries with your trainer.

If you are unsure how to manage a clinical problem it is fine to look it up (in the *BNF* or other text) in front of patients, especially if you do so with confidence. Patients are usually appreciative of your efforts to ascertain the 'latest treatment' for their condition. Electronic versions of key texts (e.g. *The Oxford Textbook of Medicine*) and clinical decision support software (e.g. Mentor) and the internet, if available, can also be helpful mid-consultation, but you will need to spend some time familiarizing yourself in how to use them.

Mid-surgery you can always ask your trainer or other staff member and afterwards you can liaise with your hospital and pharmacy colleagues as needed.* Tell the patient you will contact them and do not forget to do so.

* See Asking for help, p. 76.

'Bread and butter' medicine

While this includes some relatively straightforward problems, such as urinary tract infections and contraception, other conditions such as nappy rash and joint pains are likely to cause problems for the new registrar. They are rarely dealt with in hospitals, and generally ignored at medical school, so you will be on a steep learning curve initially. The *BNF*, in particular, and books on clinical general practice are very useful here together with experience, tutorials, home reading and MCQ practice.

Psychosocial problems

These crop up frequently in surgeries either overtly, for example as requests for housing letters or referrals for counselling, or covertly as medically unexplained symptoms. Even in cases you believe are entirely psychological, it is worth trying to exclude physical causes initially.

The impact of social circumstances and mental health on general health will be a recurring theme of many surgeries throughout your career. The 'worried well' (often affluent and well-educated middle classes) can be as challenging as impoverished, minority and refugee groups.

Arrange a tutorial on the recognition and management of depression in all its guises early in your year. You will see a lot of it.

As the year goes on you will develop skills in:

- picking up the hidden agenda, for example repeated attendance for 'minor problems' that may reflect underlying depression
- recognizing and managing somatic complaints, (physical manifestations of psychological problems)
- illness associated with secondary gain, (benefits of the sick role which consciously or unconsciously keeps people ill)
- addressing your own personal boundaries, limitations and prejudices.

You will need to include a consultation with a significant psychological or social dimension for the MRCGP exam video.

Chronic diseases

GPs manage a number of chronic diseases either alone or shared with a hospital specialist. Some practices organize specific clinics for asthma, diabetes and coronary heart disease, which allow for continuity of care for the patient while reducing some of the burden on secondary care. Many clinics are run by practice nurses with GP support using practice protocols based on national or local evidence-based guidelines. Make sure you have an opportunity to participate in any such clinics run in your practice. Familiarize yourself with the computer templates and prompts used.* The *BNF* has a wealth of information on chronic disease management including some national guidelines.

* See Data Entry, p. 121.

Acquire a few patients with chronic diseases for follow-up throughout your year; they provide an ideal opportunity to develop an on-going relationship whilst monitoring clinical progress.

Health promotion

Although this forms a large part of the practice nurse remit, you should also make use of every opportunity in routine surgeries to discuss the big 'five':

- smoking
- alcohol
- diet
- exercise
- sexual health.

Check and document blood pressure, BMI, contraception, sexual health promotion, smear and vaccination due dates. Use patient information leaflets (PILs), which may be available on computer, to reinforce your advice. Always document any advice and leaflets you give.

Emergencies in general practice

Your experience of these will depend very much on where you practice, but emergencies are much less common in the community than in hospitals, so you do risk losing your skills. Make notes of your well-learned hospital management while they are still fresh in your mind.

Your medical bag and the surgery drug cupboard should be well stocked to cover basic emergencies.†

† See Your medical bag, p. 64.

You may well have to deal with emergencies alone (in the surgery or on a visit) without the luxury of a helpful nurse. You may also have to contend with an interested lay audience, so it is useful to develop a systematic approach (*Box 9.1*).

Box 9.1   An approach to dealing with medical emergencies in general practice

- Do not panic
- Summon help (use the alarm button if you are in the surgery)
- Ensure someone calls for an ambulance and give them an idea of the diagnosis
- Assume control of the situation
- Delegate where possible
- Take time to assess the clinical situation fully: go through a history from the patient or witness, and examine the patient calmly where appropriate.
- Institute appropriate management, which may involve anything from CPR to doing nothing until an ambulance arrives
- Always wait with the patient if an ambulance is needed or ensure they are not left alone until fully recovered
- Take time to inform relatives
- Document the incident fully in the medical record
- Debrief with your trainer
- Discuss the case at practice 'critical incident' meetings if appropriate

---

What to do when you don't know what to do

Vague presentations that do not fit a clear clinical picture (e.g. tired all the time, pain all over) are prevalent in general practice. Sometimes it can be illuminating simply to ask the patient what they are worried about, or what help they want from you: ' What is it you were hoping I can do?' Otherwise buy some time by organizing some limited simple investigations (e.g. FBC, ESR/CRP, urinalysis or what else seems appropriate) and arrange a review with these results. Normal tests may well be reassuring for both you and the patient and may also allow a hidden agenda to surface. Do not hesitate to seek advice from your colleagues.

DIFFICULT CONSULTATIONS

Not all consultations go smoothly and there will be days when you are simply not on top form and have a run of difficult consultations. Do not worry – it happens to us all.

Occasionally you will feel pressurized into management you are not comfortable with, such as issuing a prescription for benzodiazepines, or referring when you deem it unnecessary. If you feel a request is inappropriate then explain why. Evidence-based medicine can help here. 'It is our practice policy' can also be a good get-out clause provided it really is that. Try to come to mutually acceptable compromise. Open discussion may bring up other issues and help avoid a confrontation. You may need to refer the patient back to their usual GP if you feel you cannot, or do not want to, manage the request yet they are insistent. There will be times when you have to give in so do not see this as a failing and document it in the notes ('patient insisted').

Breaking bad news

It is not uncommon to dread situations where you need to communicate an abnormal result with potentially serious consequences or other bad news. You may well be tempted to put it off, so here are a few tips to help:

- Prepare yourself by checking the clinical facts, discussing the situation with your colleagues and arranging a standby management plan before seeing the patient
- Invite the patient in for a review, perhaps by writing a (non-alarmist) letter such as: 'Your test results from … date have now come through. Would you please make an appointment to discuss them with me?' Do not be surprised if they phone you in a panic on receipt of the letter. By all means have some discussion over the phone but face-to-face contact is better if there is potentially bad news. Arrange a prompt appointment yourself and allow plenty of time
- Your patient may well suspect something is amiss already, so probe by asking them some open questions about the situation. 'Had you any thoughts about the tests and what they might show?' Give them plenty of time to air their thoughts or fears during which they may well arrive at the bad news themselves. If they do not then do not put off telling them
- Be honest, but not brutally so, and expect that they will not be able to take in much of what you say. You may need to back up your discussion with leaflets or put salient points, such as the diagnosis, in writing

- They may also go into denial, and you will have to find a balance between destroying this protective mechanism without colluding with them that nothing is wrong
- Explain the management options, including any you have set up already and ask them how they wish to go from here. They may well not be in a situation to answer immediately so do not force the point at this time
- Ask them how they feel about the situation, any specific fears they harbour and ask how you might be able to help allay these. Ensure they will have some support when they leave the surgery
- Make yourself available for further discussion and book them another appointment shortly afterwards to allow discussion of the questions that inevitably arise. Suggest that they have someone accompany them when they come again.

You may learn of a new serious diagnosis from hospital letters. A phone call or letter to the patient inviting them to see you is usually greatly appreciated.

Angry patients

There may be understandable reasons for patients to be angry such as illness, being kept waiting, or general distrust of medics based on previous experience. It is worth trying to stand back to find out the underlying cause.

Angry patients can often provoke strong feelings in you. If you find you are getting angry with a patient remember that it is often originating from them, not you.

Reflecting back to the patient calmly that you sense they are angry may allow them to express themselves more constructively. Try phrases like 'You seem very angry about this. How were you hoping I could help?' Acknowledging their discomfort, frustration or disappointment may also help. This will come with experience.

Debriefing after such consultations is essential (see below).

Defusing a potentially violent situation

If you sense a situation is getting out of hand, aim to defuse it by maintaining a calm exterior and tone of voice, however frightened you feel. Avoid rising to the patient's heightened state, particularly if you are being provoked ('call yourself a bloody doctor?'). Demonstrating respect and genuine concern for the patient may prevent the situation escalating.

If an error has been made then do not be too pompous to apologize. Acknowledging you may have been in the wrong can help avert a complaint and allows patients to see that you are human too, both in your error and in your ability to apologize: 'You sound very upset about ... I am sorry if ...'.*

If you really cannot negotiate with the patient then state firmly: 'I can hear what you are saying but I cannot help you if you continue to behave like this' and make it clear that you are 'not happy to continue the consultation in this manner'.

Put your safety first if you feel physically threatened and summon help using the panic button or by leaving the room. Do not worry if valuables are exposed. Get someone to call the police if the situation is escalating, or there has been violence or an assault.†

* See also If you have made a mistake, p. 233.

† See also Safety matters, p. 78.

Debriefing after a difficult consultation

Always take some time out before seeing your next patient otherwise they will get short shrift. Consider going to the toilet or putting the kettle on even if you are running late.‡ Discuss the situation fully with your trainer after surgery and try to see it as a learning experience. Identify how else you might have handled the situation. You may find the patient has the same effect on everyone and simply has unreasonable expectations that might be addressed in future consultations.

‡ See also Stress management strategies, Box 8.1, p. 79.

If a patient has been threatening, or there has been violence, document the event meticulously in the medical records. Ensure the patient's notes are flagged, relevant practice staff are informed and consider arrangements for future consultations in secure settings. Whether or not to report the event to the police, or even press charges, may be a consideration, and this you should discuss with your trainer.

Do not underestimate your need to debrief fully after such events. Aside from your trainer, discussion with your VTS colleagues can be helpful. You may need to seek more formal counselling, otherwise you may find both your confidence and clinical performance compromised.

DIFFICULT PATIENT TYPES

By far the largest majority of our patients are pleasant, grateful and open to medical advice. However there are a minority who are not and cause a disproportionate amount of angst for GPs. It is important to put these into perspective and not let one difficult patient cast a negative shadow over the others you see that day.

Some patients will like you and some will not, no matter how hard you try. We simply cannot please all of our patients all of the time. Do not be misled by the 'flatterers', who may want special attention from you, or conversely, the 'rejectors', who do not come back and see you. These actions may be conscious or unconscious on the part of the patient.

Some patients shop around and see every new doctor in the hope of finding the one who finally understands them. Although you might be just that doctor, you are more likely to be flavour of the month then rejected like all the rest. Looking through the notes may confirm this pattern, although some patients genuinely do not mind who they see so long as they do not have to wait long.

There are some well-recognized categories of patients (see below) which present management challenges for the GP, often with lengthy and frequent consultations. Many have deep psychological difficulties that they are unable to address or even recognize, despite reflection from an astute doctor.

Heartsinks

These patients literally make your heart sink at the prospect of a consultation with them. They include four stereotypes (*Box 9.2*).

* See Sources and further reading.

Box 9.2   Types of heartsink patients (Groves)*

- Dependent clingers
- Entitled demanders
- Manipulative help-rejectors
- Self-destructive deniers

They can be very difficult to help and can produce feelings of exasperation, depression and helplessness in the doctor, which may be a transference of how they themselves feel. Interestingly patients who are heartsinks for one GP do not necessarily produce the same reaction in another doctor. Being clear about what you can and cannot provide for them may be helpful.

Somatisers

Such patients experience and complain of physical symptoms that are medically inexplicable, and usually reflect underlying psychosocial distress that the patient cannot accept as an explanation.

They often have thick notes, wide-ranging and repeated specialist referrals and investigations with no substantial 'medical' problem found. They may also demand small-print investigations or to try all new or complementary treatments.

Management tips include:

- recognizing the pattern
- acknowledging fully the physical symptoms and the distress they cause and
- encouraging them to see the same overseeing doctor, who should limit referrals.

Frequent attenders

These, by definition, consult many more times than the average of 3.5 consultations per patient a year. They are a very mixed group, encompassing somatisers and heartsinks as well as those with multiple complex problems and physical disease. Management tips include:

- making clear problem lists
- planning regular follow-up and
- encouraging the patient to share responsibility for managing their health problems.

Manipulative patients

Some patients, particularly substance misusers, know how to 'play the system' and can be very manipulative. They may respond well to firm boundaries such as a mutual contract setting out the circumstances under which they will and will not be treated. This can help them to share some responsibility for their actions. If they do not stick to the contract they will not get what they want, so do not give in. You will develop the experience and confidence to do this as your career progresses.

Do not be put off by threats: it is *not* your fault if patients use street drugs because you would not give them Valium (or whatever they demand). Sympathize with their distress but remind them it is their choice to do so whilst you make arrangements for longer-term plans such as arranging rehabilitation.

However, we all get duped into agreeing prescriptions from time to time so give only short courses if you cannot avoid prescribing.

GIFTS FROM PATIENTS

It is delightful to receive gifts and thank you letters from grateful patients, but it is not without its problems. Be wary of the occasional patient who regularly showers you with gifts in the hope of gaining special attention. If you suspect this is the case then address it sensitively, otherwise it may hamper effective doctor–patient communication. Some gifts (such as hideous ornaments) may be difficult to refuse!

Your practice may have a policy on cash gifts; in general it is wise to refuse cash or money. Suggest instead that the patient buys something for the benefit of all the practice or donates it to charity, so have one in mind. Chocolates and alcohol received at Christmas may be divided up amongst the practice staff.

Your contract should stipulate that any gift you receive, including money or legacies, belongs to you and not the practice.

It is a good idea to keep a file or record of any gifts or letters you receive. Look through them on bad days to remind yourself of patients' appreciation.

PERSONAL QUESTIONS FROM PATIENTS

GPs vary as to how much personal information they are prepared to divulge to their patients. Enquiries about your age, residence and whether you can be called by your first name are not uncommon and can be awkward to deal with. In general, limit the information you share, particularly if you feel it could be used to your disadvantage.

GPs do become friends with their patients, particularly if they have known each other for a long time and seen children grow up, so trust your instincts. However, remember that it can be difficult to treat friends (and family) as objectively as you would your other patients and they may expect special favours from you.

SOURCES AND FURTHER READING

1. Risdale L. *Evidence-based General Practice, a Critical Reader*, Saunders, 1996.
2. Neighbour R. *The Inner Consultation.* Petroc Press, 1999.
3. Tate P. *The Doctor's Communication Handbook*, 3rd edition, Radcliffe Medical Press, 2001.
4. Pendleton D. et al. *The Consultation.* Oxford University Press, 1984.
5. Balint M. *The Doctor, His Patient and the Illness.* Churchill Livingstone, 2000.
6. Groves J.E. Taking care of the hateful patient. *New Engl. J. Med.* **298:** 883–887, 1978.
7. Gill D., Sharpe M. Frequent consulters in general practice: a systematic review of studies of prevalence, associations and outcome. *J. Psychosom. Res.* **47**(2): 115–130, 1999.

10
Prescribing

INTRODUCTION

> *You have legal and clinical responsibility for any prescription you sign. Do not sign any you are not entirely confident about, particularly if they are initiated or generated by someone else.*

Prescribing in primary care is a hugely expensive and complex area of health provision. In 1999 prescribing throughout the NHS accounted for 13% of the entire NHS budget, nearly £7 billion a year.

Each consultation need not end with a prescription ('script'), but many do. An estimated 69% of patients consulting GPs in 1998 received a prescription. A recommendation for an over-the-counter (OTC) preparation may be more appropriate and can save money both for patients who pay for their prescriptions and the NHS.

Early in your GP registrar year you will need to concentrate on matching appropriate medication to condition, but your awareness of prescribing protocols, generic prescribing and drug costs should increase as the year progresses.

Further prescribing tips are given in Chapter 7: Practical Preparations for Consulting, Drugs for your bag, p. 66, Chapter 11: Medical Records and Computers, Prescribing on the computer, p. 121 and Chapter 18: Out-of-hours, Using drugs out-of-hours, p. 181.

GOOD PRESCRIBING PRACTICE

It is essential to adhere to good prescribing practice (*Box 10.1*). Medication errors account for a large number of complaints and medico-legal claims. The commonest mistakes to make are:

- wrong dosage
- right drug prescribed to the wrong patient
- inappropriate repeat prescribing (see later)
- new drug interacts with existing medication
- inappropriate medication
- failure to monitor treatment
- failure of communication between doctor and patient.

Make sure your patient understands what they are being prescribed, what side effects to look out for and what adverse effects to report. It is useful to give patients a list of their current medication.

Aim for evidence-based, cost-effective and safe prescribing with a fully counselled patient. Keep up with the latest evidence-based guidelines, use drug information sources freely (see end of chapter) and develop a good relationship with your local pharmacist.

WRITING PRESCRIPTIONS

GP prescriptions are made on the FP10 form or its computer equivalent FP10 comp. These are issued to the practice by the health authority and bear the GP principal's name, prescribing number, surgery address and telephone number so all prescriptions can be traced.

Named principals sign their own allocated prescriptions. Registrars and non-principals prescribe under their trainer's or another principal's name. Add your name in block capitals to your signature so the pharmacist can identify you as the prescriber should queries arise.

Box 10.1 Good prescribing practice

- Consider carefully whether the treatment is really indicated
- Always carry and consult with a current *BNF*
- Prescribe safely, so check specifically for:
  - known allergies
  - interactions and polypharmacy
  - pregnancy and breast-feeding.
- Prescribe generically unless medically inappropriate (*Box 10.5*)
- Avoid combination formulations (except oral contraception and HRT)
- Abide by existing practice formularies or prescribing protocols
- Be aware of maximum duration of treatment per prescription
- Limit the amount of drug you issue for known drug users or where you doubt the genuineness of request
- Document all treatment fully in the medical record with review arrangements
- Document medication reviews
- Update prescribing records following home visits, out-of-hours contacts and specialist reviews
- Develop an awareness of drug costs (although cheaper is not always better)

Accurate completion of prescriptions is detailed below (*Box 10.2*) and your computer-prescribing program will also give you helpful prompts. The pharmacist will contact you if there are errors on the prescription.

Familiarize yourself with the information on the reverse of the FP10 as you may occasionally need to complete this on behalf of your patients.

Prescriptions are valid for 6 months from the date of issue except those for controlled drugs, which are valid for 13 weeks. An estimated 14.5% of prescriptions are not cashed in at all. Advise patients to destroy any unused prescriptions.

Reducing prescription fraud

Prescription theft and fraud is estimated to cost the NHS £15 million a year in England and Wales alone, so be vigilant to help reduce this (*Box 10.3*). All FP10s are now numbered so you may have to sign out and account for all prescriptions you use. Your practice or health authority may want to keep wasted prescriptions.

Box 10.2 Accurate completion of prescriptions

- Use indelible ink
- Patient's full name and address, plus age (essential if 12 or under) or date of birth
- Medicine name
- Medicine formulation (tablet, capsule, soluble, syrup, suppository, cream, patch, etc.)
- Route (p.o., p.r., p.v., sublingual, buccal, topical, transdermal, etc.)
- Dose (write out micrograms or nanograms in full)
- Frequency
- Total quantity or duration of course
- Your signature (and print your name if not your prescription)
- Date
  o.d. = once daily; b.d. = twice; t.d.s. = three times; q.d.s. = four times; p.r.n. = as required (pharmacists prefer specific instructions); o.p. = standard pack size or tube of cream

---

Information obtained from, www.BNF.org.

Box 10.3   Reducing prescription fraud, tampering and theft

- Circle the quantity issued, or duration of course
- Rule a diagonal line though any blank space (computer may do so automatically)
- Countersign/initial any alterations
- Keep prescriptions out of sight (in consulting room, car, at reception)
- Keep prescriptions in a locked drawer
- Take few prescriptions on visits

Information obtained from, www.BNF.org

OPTIMIZING PATIENT COMPLIANCE

Counsel your patient fully, particularly when starting new drugs (*Box 10.4*). Many packaged medicines have clear patient information leaflets, but patients can be put off by the comprehensive list of possible side effects. You may need to put this into perspective for them.

Ensure your patient knows when and how to get a repeat prescription (see below) and when to come for review. Try to synchronize the due dates for each drug for those on multiple medications.

GENERIC PRESCRIBING

Prescribing by drug name rather than proprietary (brand) name is cost-effective, encourages consistency and is used as a measure of good prescribing. When presented with a generic prescription, pharmacists are not obliged to dispense a particular brand. You should explain to the patient that, on occasion, they may get a different looking drug or even a different name on the package but this should not affect their treatment. It may be counter-productive to emphasize the cost difference to patients. There are a few exceptions where it is medically necessary to prescribe a particular brand (*Box 10.5*).

LONG-TERM MEDICATION

To ensure safe prescribing for patients on long-term treatments, systematic reviews of medication and a foolproof repeat prescribing system are essential.

Box 10.4   Prescribing: counselling the patient

- Make clear:
  - the purpose of any medicine prescribed – is it a cure, symptom relief or prevention?
  - intended duration of treatment
  - review arrangements
  - specific drug monitoring if appropriate.
- Warn about:
  - common side effects
  - significant interactions
  - potential for dependency and tolerance
  - other specific instructions.
- Give written instructions for complex or changing regimes, e.g. reducing steroids
- Explain the practice repeat prescribing system

The medication review

Ideally this should be undertaken by the doctor who knows the patient best. Devise a systematic approach to these reviews (*Box 10.6*) and incorporate them opportunistically into your routine consultations and daytime home visits. Document the review in the medical record.

Box 10.5   Exceptions to generic prescribing

Drugs with a narrow therapeutic index
- Lithium
- Cyclosporin

Modified release preparations (where different formulations give different bioavailability)
- Theophylline/aminophylline
- Diltiazem/nifedipine
- Anticonvulsants

Others
- Most oral contraceptives
- Some HRT preparations
- Combination medications (though generally not recommended anyway)

Box 10.6 Systematic approach to medication review

- Is the patient taking the medications you think they are taking?
- Review the original and continuing requirement for each drug and dose:
  - Is it still appropriate?
  - Is it effective?
  - Is it the most cost-effective?
  - Is it being taken properly and are directions clear?
- Do they understand the purpose of the drugs?
- Are they happy to continue taking them?
- Ask specifically about:
  - side effects (consider dose or drug changes if significant)
  - alcohol intake
  - other non-prescribed medications also taken (OTC, herbal and homeopathic treatments) and check interactions with these where known.
- Institute relevant monitoring tests (including blood tests/BP) and ensure the patient understands the need for and frequency of these
- Chase up results and notify the patient of any necessary drug changes
- Clarify with the patient, with written instructions if necessary, and document:
  - current regime, including new drugs and whether they are additions or substitutes
  - changes made at review
  - tests initiated with results
  - arrangement for next review.

Patients under shared hospital and GP care

Department of Health guidelines stipulate that where care is shared between hospital doctors and GPs, the legal responsibility for prescribing lies with the doctor who signs the prescription. *

* Adapted from the BNF at, www.BNF.org.

Essentially the prescriber is responsible for reviewing the treatment. GPs often have to issue repeat prescriptions after hospital reviews and so must ensure that written documentation and test results are available from the hospital visits before prescribing. Chasing up such information can be time-consuming but is essential for patient safety.

* See Clinical Post, p. 158.

Medication changes should also be recorded in the prescribing and medical record, and review dates amended when hospital letters are dealt with.* Messages can be added to the medical record and computer prescribing record, for example 'under anticoagulant clinic, last reviewed ...' or 'TFTs adequately replaced at endocrine clinic on ...' to avoid duplication of tests.

Repeat prescribing

> **Repeat prescribing lends itself to mistakes, complaints and litigation so take rigorous clinical care when signing each prescription.**

The practice's repeat prescribing system allows prescriptions to be issued without the need for a face-to-face consultation each time. This has been revolutionized by computerization, although a few practices still write out all their repeats by hand. The computer also generates a list of repeat medication that can be used for future requests and to remind patients of review dates.

Practice repeat prescribing protocol

All practices should have a written protocol that is reviewed at least annually (*Box 10.7*). Familiarize yourself with the system so you can educate your patients accordingly. As the new person in the practice you, and your audit, are in a good position to identify and improve on any flaws in the current system.

Dealing with repeat prescription requests

Repeat prescriptions may be generated by a trained staff member, but must be checked and signed by a doctor. As a GP registrar you should not be expected to sign the repeat prescriptions early in your year. If and when you are involved you should be fully supervised.

Check all the details on the prescription. If queries arise, access the medical record, or contact the patient to satisfy yourself that the prescription is appropriate. Refuse to sign if you are not sure and ask the patient to make an appointment.

You may need to pass unsigned prescriptions back to the partner who knows the patient best.

If a review is due you may agree to prescribe a short supply but make it clear that the patient must come in for a review with their GP before the next prescription is issued.

Box 10.7   Repeat prescribing protocol

Should clarify:

Submission of prescription requests
- Written, usually with 48 hours notice
- Faxes or e-mails acceptable but generally not phone requests

Access to prescriptions
- Collection at surgery or in liaison with local pharmacist (may arrange repeats automatically or even deliver)
- By post if patient supplies self-addressed envelope

Maximum quantity/duration per prescription
- Often 1–3 months
- 6 months for oral contraception/HRT may be permissible

Frequency of review
- For example, 1–2 months for antidepressants, 6 months for oral contraception/HRT

Medication unsuitable for repeats (so a face-to-face consultation essential)
- For example, night sedation, antidepressants in the suicidal, NSAIDs in the elderly

Fail-safe system (computer very helpful here)
- Specific review period or dates should be entered and observed
- Heed computer warnings of over- or under-use of medication
- Prescriptions not to be issued if review overdue until patient seen
- Computer messages may be added, e.g. 'No more DF118 until seen', with date and your initials

---

Reception staff will be responsible for sending out prescriptions or leaving them for collection, usually in an indexed box. You may be asked by reception staff to sign *ad hoc* repeat prescriptions for patients who 'cannot wait' (going on holiday, etc.). Always adhere to your good prescribing practice even when under pressure.

PRESCRIBING IN SPECIFIC CASES

See also the relevant pages in the *BNF*, www.BNF.org.

For the elderly

Take care with drug doses, reduce polypharmacy where possible and be alert to interactions. Try to avoid prescribing drugs with the potential for sedation and confusion. Prescribe very small quantities of drugs where you feel the drug is indicated but are concerned about potential adverse effects. Review the patient and do not put the drug on 'repeat', e.g. for NSAIDs.

Use every opportunity to review medication, including home visits. Encourage patients to return obsolete or date-expired medicines to their pharmacist. You may even remove them yourself, but only with the patient's permission.

Dosset boxes can help to organize those on multiple medications, but access to the compartments may be difficult and drug or dose changes can be complicated to institute. The pharmacist or district nurse will make up the dosset box on a regular basis, but this in itself does not ensure compliance.

In pregnancy and breast-feeding

Always check if a woman is, or might be, pregnant or is breast-feeding before prescribing and comply with advice in the *BNF* appendices. Manufacturers may advise against use in pregnancy and breast-feeding because of lack of evidence on safe usage.

Anxiety often arises in women who may have taken drugs before realizing they are pregnant. In some cases you may need to liaise with your hospital drug information service, the Regional and District Medicines Information Service (details in *BNF*) or even the manufacturers for advice.

For children

Prescribe according to any available paediatric formulary. You may need to use unlicensed medicines or licensed medicines for unlicensed purposes (see below) when prescribing in children. In such cases the parent/carer and child, where appropriate, should be fully informed and agreeable to the treatment.

Always check doses even for those drugs you think you know well. Most doses are given for age ranges or weight. In primary care you will rarely need to prescribe according to body surface area but there is a helpful conversion table at the back of the *BNF*. Get a colleague to double-check any dose calculations you make.

Advise parents of the indications for the medicine and of potential side effects, and remind them of safe storage of all medicines. Check for family history of severe penicillin allergy before prescribing for the first time.

Prescribe sugar-free formulations where available and avoid tablets or i.m. injections. The standard 5 ml medicine spoon is supplied where the dose is a multiple of 5 ml, otherwise a medicine syringe will be supplied by the pharmacist. Syringes are particularly useful for 'difficult' children. Advise parents to place the syringe between the cheek and gum margin, not directly on the tongue, with the child held at 45 degrees. Drugs should not be added to bottles or feeds.

All prescriptions for children under 16, or under 18 in full-time education, are free.

Antibiotics

Before prescribing antibiotics check for history of:

- **allergy**
- **pregnancy**
- **breast-feeding**
- **oral contraceptive use.**

Follow local guidelines and be aware of local resistance patterns, for example for UTIs.

Be consistent in your refusal of antibiotics for the treatment of simple upper respiratory infections. Explain why they are not appropriate and back it up with written advice and OTC recommendations. This may take longer than issuing a prescription, but it pays dividends in the long run. If necessary come to a compromise and issue a prescription to be used should symptoms deteriorate within a specified time.

Prescribing over the phone

Prescriptions, with the exception of controlled drugs, can be telephoned through to a local pharmacist for collection by patients. This can be useful out-of-hours or following a telephone consultation, but should only be undertaken if you are confident of your decision to initiate or continue treatment without the need for a face-to-face consultation. Antibiotics should not be prescribed over the phone except in exceptional circumstances. Send the written prescription to the pharmacist promptly.

Homeopathic and herbal medicines

Some of these treatments are available on FP10s. Unless you are specifically trained you may not be happy to prescribe, so make this clear to the patient. Suggest they see one of the partners or refer them to a homeopathically qualified doctor.

Some herbal treatments have significant side effects and interactions (e.g. St. John's Wort and the combined oral contraceptive pill) so advise patients not to assume that natural treatments are harmless.

Controlled drugs

Marked CD in the *BNF*, controlled drugs include the familiar opioids and barbiturates. Controlled drug prescriptions must be written in full by hand in indelible ink. You must include:

- patient's name and address
- drug form
- dose, strength and the total quantity in words and figures
- your address, signature and hand-written date.

Computer-printed prescriptions for controlled drugs are not accepted, but you may write out the details on a blank FP10 comp.

Pharmacists will phone you to reissue the prescription if it is not completed accurately as they are not legally permitted to dispense the drugs in such situations. (They often make allowances for mistakes on prescriptions for non-CD drugs, dispense the medication then send back the prescription for correction.)

The use of controlled drugs is governed by the Misuse of Drugs Act 1971 and the Misuse of Drugs Regulations amended in 1985. Registered medical practitioners are allowed to 'possess and supply CDs when acting in a professional capacity' with the exception of schedule 1 drugs (*Box 10.8*). Doctors can be prosecuted for contravention of any of these regulations.

Controlled drugs must be kept in a locked compartment or receptacle and must be in a locked case if left in a locked car boot. The practice must keep a register to record supply and use of CDs that the police or Home Office inspectors have a right to inspect every 2 years.

Advise patients taking CDs and going abroad that they may require a specific licence from the Home Office, particularly if taking sizeable quantities of Schedule 2 and 3 drugs. Doctors carrying CDs abroad accompanying patients may also need a licence.

> **Box 10.8   Controlled drug schedules (Misuse of Drugs Regulations 1985)**
>
> Schedule 1: cannabis/LSD – no therapeutic use (except research)
> Schedule 2: opiates and major stimulants
> Schedule 3: most barbiturates and some minor stimulants
> Schedule 4: benzodiazepines
> Schedule 5: CDs combined with other drugs with minimal risk of abuse

Prescribing in the treatment of addiction

A special licence is required to prescribe heroin, cocaine or morphine in the treatment of addiction. For these, and methadone, the special blue prescription form FP10 MDA (GP10 in Scotland) should be used. Drug misusers no longer have to be registered with the Home Office, but doctors should report cases to the regional centre of the National Drugs Treatment Monitoring System (details in the *BNF*).

Many practices will register drug-dependent patients for primary health-care services, but may leave CD prescribing to the local Drug Dependency Unit. You will need to get specific training if you are to prescribe methadone.

Requests for drugs that you suspect are being used as alternatives to street drugs, typically benzodiazepines and opioids, can be difficult to manage.* Be guided by practice policy and ask for advice. If you do agree to prescribe these drugs, limit supplies to a few days only.

* See also Manipulative patients, p. 93.

PAYING FOR MEDICINES

The patient

Prescription charges and exemptions

NHS prescription charges are set by government and increased most years. Ninety percent of all prescriptions issued in 1998 were exempt from charges for medical, maternity and social reasons or on the grounds of age (*Box 10.9*). Pharmacists are increasingly vigilant in checking for evidence of eligibility for exemption from charges. All contraception is available free in the UK.

Medical and maternity exemption certificates are issued by the health authority following the submission of form FP92A (for medical

Box 10.9   Prescription charge exemptions

See reverse of FP10
- Aged under 16
- Aged 16, 17, 18 and in full-time education
- Aged 60 or over
- Holder of maternity exemption certificate
- Holder of medical exemption certificate (see below)
- Holder of prepayment certificate
- Holder of war pension exemption certificate
- Named on HC2 charges certificate (entitled to help with health costs)
- Receiving:
  - Income Support
  - Income-based Job Seeker's Allowance
  - full Working Families Tax Credit
  - Disabled Person's Tax Credit.
- Prescribed contraception

Quoted from form FP10. Crown copyright material is reproduced with the permission of the Controller of HMSO and the Queen's Printer for Scotland.

conditions – *Box 10.10*) or FW8 (for maternity cases). These should be available in the surgery, completed by the patient, countersigned by the GP confirming the condition then forwarded to the health authority that issues the certificate.

Holders of medical exemption certificates are entitled to free medicines for all conditions, not only the qualifying one. Prepayment certificates can work out cheaper for patients who require regular prescriptions but are not exempt from charges.

Over-the-counter medicines

Medicines are classified according to their availability to the public, generally on grounds of safety and tolerability (*Box 10.11*).
A large number of medicines are available over-the-counter without prescription and it is always worth checking in the *BNF* when you prescribe. The Proprietary Association of Great Britain publishes an annual directory of such medicines. The pharmacist's role as health advisor continues to expand along with the list of P and OTC medicines, with the intention of encouraging self-care and reducing GP contacts. Patients exempt from charges or requiring a large quantity of a non-prescription medicine may still request prescriptions.

Box 10.11   Classification of medicines

PoM: prescription-only medication
P: pharmacy – can be sold from pharmacists
GSL: general sales list – can be sold from shops and supermarkets

Private prescriptions

Private prescriptions can only be issued to NHS patients for medication that cannot be prescribed on an FP10. Although some drugs available on FP10 may be cheaper on private prescription, GPs are not actually allowed to offer a private prescription alternative to their patients.

There are some prescription-only medicines in occasional use, marked NHS in the *BNF*, which cannot be prescribed on an NHS prescription. Where patients insist on such items, and you feel the request is justified, you can issue a private prescription. Warn the patient that they will have to meet the full cost of the drug together with a pharmacist's dispensing fee, so do not quote them the *BNF* price, which is discounted for NHS use only.

Such drugs include:

- sildenafil (Viagra) for certain patient groups
- mefloquine (Lariam) for malarial prophylaxis (but not treatment of established cases)
- 'blacklisted' benzodiazepines.

The NHS does not support the prescription of 'just in case drugs' such as antibiotics for foreign travel, so you will need to prescribe privately if you agree to such requests.

Patients who have been seen in the private sector and issued with a private prescription often ask for these to be converted to NHS prescriptions as their insurance will not cover drug costs. Discuss these occasional cases with your trainer or another GP.

Private prescriptions can be issued by computer or by hand and must include your professional address and GMC number. They can be used to buy in drugs to stock your doctor's bag.

The health service

PACT – Prescribing Analysis and Cost data

PACT data is issued every 3 months to all GP principals by the Prescription Pricing Authority (PPA) which processes all dispensed NHS prescriptions. It provides summaries of individual GPs' and practice prescribing with information on the number of individual items and costs of the prescriptions dispensed (not issued). Local and national comparisons are provided together with data for the previous year.

Drugs are divided into the main six *BNF* therapeutic groups and the 20 leading prescriptions in the practice are identified. Practices can use this information to audit their prescribing.

Look through your trainer's PACT report in a tutorial. It will focus you on just how expensive drugs are and it could be the basis of an MRCGP question.

Prescribing incentive schemes

Such schemes, run by health authorities or PCG/PCTs, offer financial rewards to practices that fulfil certain 'good practice' prescribing criteria. Such criteria vary from region to region and from year to year but may include:

- high percentage of generic prescriptions
- low percentage of drugs known to be of limited therapeutic value
- ratio of bronchodilator to steroid inhalers prescribed
- NSAIDs prescribed from a locally approved list.

Find out how your practice is involved and try to help prescribe in line with local policy.

High-cost medication

Some expensive specialist drugs are initiated in secondary care and GPs are then asked to continue prescribing them. GPs are not obliged to prescribe if they are not willing to accept the clinical responsibility involved. This is particularly relevant for new specialist treatments where the GP may feel insufficiently experienced to prescribe.

Such treatments, which include fertility drugs, erythropoietin injections and enteral nutritional supplements, may cost thousands of pounds per patient per year. Your practice should have a policy on such prescribing based on local recommendations. As a GP registrar it should not be up to you to decide whether or not to prescribe such drugs. Discuss such cases with your trainer or other partner.

GPs agreeing to prescribe high-cost medicines may need to inform the prescribing advisor for their PCG/PCT or health authority to ensure these items are excluded from the annual practice drug costs.

DRUG SAFETY ISSUES

Reporting adverse drug reactions (ADRs)

Remember to report adverse reactions to the Medicines Control Agency using the Yellow Card system at the back of the *BNF*. You should report (for any therapeutic agent, including self-medication and herbal products):

- any reaction from new drugs (marked ▼ in the BNF)
- severe reactions from established drugs even if a well-recognized reaction.

Drug and product liability

Drug manufacturers are liable for their products under the Consumer Protection Act 1987 and patients can claim compensation from them should they suffer injury as a result of specific drug use. To avoid this

DRUG INFORMATION SOURCES

	WRITTEN MATERIAL
The *BNF*	• Excellent source of information on clinical management as well as drug use
	• Always use the current version: issued March and September.
	• Read essential information in the front and appendices
	• Useful phone numbers inside front cover
	• Directory of drug manufacturers at the back
	• Electronic version available (eBNF) and on-line at BNF.org
OTC (Over-the-counter Directory) (Proprietary Association of Great Britain)	• Useful guide to save you issuing prescriptions and to save money for your patients
Practice or PCG/ PCT prescribing protocol or formulary	• Usually based on local prescribing guidance
	• Some exceptions are likely in practice
Drug and Therapeutics Bulletin	• Excellent and sensible evidence-based assessment of common therapeutic issues
	• Essential for day-to-day practice and MRCGP exam
MeReC Bulletin	• Regular bulletin providing clear, concise evaluated information on medicines and prescribing-related issues
	• Published by National Prescribing Centre and funded by NICE
	• Available on-line at npc.co.uk
Drug Tariff	• NHS publication supplied to practices and pharmacists outlining all brands, clinical supplies and equipment available on the NHS
	• Useful for troublesome prescriptions for stoma bags, dressings, catheters, etc.

SERVICES AND ORGANIZATIONS

Local pharmacists	• Often underused resource • Normally happy to offer advice so keep phone number handy
Hospital pharmacists and drug information service.	• Helpful for queries, particularly on new drugs and interactions
PCG/PCT prescribing advisor	• Pharmacists employed by PCG/PCT to advise on local prescribing issues • Help with practice audit
Regional and district medicines information services	• Phone numbers inside front cover of the *BNF* • Provide information on any aspect of drug therapy
Local poisons unit	• Phone number inside front cover of the *BNF* • First contact for acute overdose/poisoning incidents
Pharmacy at the Royal London Homeopathic Hospital	• Provide advice on homeopathic treatment including interactions with orthodox medicines
Drug companies	• Index of all manufacturers at back of *BNF* • Contact drug information departments for information on their individual products
National Prescribing Centre (NPC)	• NHS organization promoting high-quality cost-effective prescribing
Prescription Pricing Authority (PPA)	• NHS 'special health authority' • Provides feedback to prescribers, via PACT, and to Department of Health • Sets pricing arrangements for paying pharmacists and prescribing practices

liability falling to you as the GP, you must ensure the patient is fully informed about the appropriate use of the drug and keep adequate records documenting:

- date of prescription
- nature of illness
- tests to establish diagnosis
- quantity prescribed
- warnings of side effects
- problems experienced by the patient while taking the drug.

You must document clearly the dose, batch number and expiry date of any drugs or injections you administer yourself.

Prescribing unlicensed drugs

Drugs sold in the UK must have a product licence (Marketing Authorization) that confirms quality, safety and efficiency.

There may be occasions when unlicensed drugs can be prescribed, or licensed drugs prescribed for indications outside their licence. In such cases the patient or parent must be fully informed that the drug is unlicensed and that all actions and side effects may not be known. The prescribing doctor (and not the manufacturer) must be prepared to take full responsibility for all the side effects. Such drugs may be available from the manufacturer or licensed importer on a 'named patient' only basis.

You may need to seek advice from your colleagues or medical protection organization in such situations.

SOURCES AND FURTHER READING

1. Current *BNF* (www.BNF.org)
2. RCGP. Information Sheet no. 10. *Prescribing in General Practice*, September 2000.
3. Medical Protection Society. *Managing the Risks in General Practice.* MPS, 2001.
4. Royal College of Paediatrics and Child Health. *The use of unlicensed medicines or licensed medicines for unlicensed application in paediatric practice.* Policy statement from RCPCH and Neonatal and Paediatric Pharmacists Group, February 2000.
5. National Prescribing Centre website, www.npc.co.uk
6. Prescription Pricing Authority website, www.ppa.org.uk
7. Medicines Control Agency website, www.open.gov.uk/mca/mcahome.htm
8. Drug and Therapeutics Bulletin website, www.which.net/health/dtb

11
Medical records and computers

INTRODUCTION

Processing and protecting information about patients is an integral part of a GP's work. The computer has an ever-increasing role in health-care, and GPs are often ahead of their hospital colleagues in the use of IT in their day-to-day work. As most practices use computers for some, if not all, of the patients' medical record, this chapter considers the medical record and computer together.

MEDICAL RECORDS

Whether in paper or electronic format medical records are essential for continuity of patient care and provide good medico-legal protection. Lost notes can slow up your surgery and impair good medical practice. Do not do a consultation without them if possible.

NHS medical records belong to the health authority and neither the GP nor the patient. A doctor only has the legal right to use the notes to provide on-going clinical care.

Documenting the consultation

> **Always write full and clear notes, particularly following a difficult consultation and ensure the date and time are documented.**

The test of an adequate medical record is that it enables you to reconstruct the consultation without reference to memory. GPs vary as to how much information they record and whether they complete records during or after the consultation. As a registrar it is probably best to complete the medical record after each consultation. Try not to leave this until the end of the surgery, even if you are running late, as you will forget important details.

The acronym 'SOAP' can be used to structure the consultation findings in the notes (*Box 11.1*).

Documenting the consultation can take several minutes so allow for this in the time you allocate for each consultation. Your notes will become slicker with experience and time pressure, but should always include a sensible minimum of information. You should:

- document relevant negative findings to show you actively considered them
- avoid writing derogatory comments about the patient, their relatives or colleagues

Box 11.1 Documenting consultations: SOAP

S Subjective What the patient tells you/history
O Objective Your examination findings
A Assessment Your working diagnosis/problem title
P Plan Your management: investigations,
           referrals, treatment and follow-up

- avoid the excessive use of abbreviations
- record any health promotion advice you give, even as a throwaway comment (essential for audit and clinical governance)
- document extra consultations such as phone consultations, out-of-hours consultations, discussions with hospital specialists about patients and opinions you give on patients the nurse asks you to 'pop in and see for a moment'.

Taking care of medical records

Respect patients' medical records! Do not leave them lying around where other patients could read them or leave your computer screen showing details of your previous patient. Ideally paper records should not be removed from the surgery, except for home visits, although occasionally you will have to take them home for paperwork (when you are a principal!). Never leave notes in your car.

Reception staff should be aware of the importance of confidentiality, accurate filing and the use of a reliable tracer system.

Disclosure of medical information from the medical records to a third party is covered in detail in Chapter 23: Guidance for Good Professional Practice, Disclosing medical information, p. 229.

Amending medical records

Never go back and rewrite notes at a later date.

Records should only be amended if the information is inaccurate, misleading or incomplete. If you need to make changes then make it clear you are doing so by adding a note that you should date and sign. Should a patient disagree with an entry then it can be amended (not removed) with a dated statement from the patient to that effect. Do not make any changes that could later be interpreted as an intention to mislead. Computer programs are able to trace changes and deletions made to patients' notes so ensure you always log on correctly and do not allow others to use your terminal without changing to their username and password first.

Patients cannot dictate what information goes into their notes; it is up to the doctor to decide what is relevant for the clinical care of the patient. You may need to explain this to patients who ask you to omit certain information from their notes where you feel it would be clinically inappropriate to do so. If you do enter the information and are subsequently challenged by the patient then be prepared to justify your decision.

In certain clinical situations, however, it may be appropriate to negotiate with the patient whether to exclude certain information, such as a negative HIV test. Future disclosure of clinical information to a third party, particularly insurers, can have adverse non-medical implications for the patient.

Patient access to medical records

Under the Data Protection Act (1998) patients are allowed access to their entire medical record, unless:

- the doctor feels disclosure of information would cause *serious* harm to their mental or physical health or
- information about a third party would be revealed without their consent.

Bear in mind the following points that should be explained to patients wishing to see their records:

- requests should be made in writing to the practice
- no reason is needed
- the practice must supply the patient, or someone authorized on their behalf, with copies of the relevant notes within 40 days of the request unless there are good reasons to deny access (see above)
- explanations must be given if information is not easy to understand (e.g. medical abbreviations) either by appointment or in writing
- all written requests for access to notes should be date-stamped and kept with copies of the information disclosed, separate from the notes.

If a patient asks to see their records there and then, you should discuss it with your trainer. Although the act does not give patients the right to inspect their records straight away, if both the note-holder and patient agree, and the above exemptions do not apply, then you may let them have immediate access.

The Data Protection Act also covers issues on protecting patient information.

COMPUTERS

Most training practices are now computerized and many aim to be 'paper-lean'. Practices and GPs vary in the extent to which they use their computers (*see Box 11.2*), but most computerized practices use

---

Box 11.2   Potential uses of the computer in general practice

Look at the main menu on your computer package

Patient management
- Medical records
- Past history
- Medical summary including new patient registration check
- Consultation entries
- Results
- Chronic disease management templates
- Diary due-dates
- Prescribing
- Word-processing
- Referral letters
- Scanned documents
- Clinical protocols and guidelines

Practice management
- Appointments system
- Practice profile/demographics
- Practice accounts

Databases
- Practice phone directory
- eBNF
- Patient information leaflets
- Medical decision support software, e.g. Mentor

Communications
- Internal and external e-mail
- Links to hospital pathology laboratory/radiology
- Links to health authority for claims
- NHSnet
- Internet

Research and education
- Patient searches
- Audit
- Statistical analysis
- Medline/other search
- On-line journals/circulars

---

their systems for repeat prescribing and clinical records. Medical records on hard disk are less likely to get lost than their paper equivalents and are more accessible for audit. There are, however, significant confidentiality implications and system failures can cause havoc.

Several GP software packages are available with training, upgrades and helplines. No package is perfect and their illogicalities cause frequent frustration. Most packages allow you to enter data as free text and also in response to fixed prompts, which are coded and can be easily traced for audit and research purposes.

Technophobes should make an effort to embrace these tools. If you are lucky enough to have your own individual PC in your room use it for word-processing, external communications and your written work for summative assessment.

Training

Entering information on the computer during surgeries will slow you down to start with so make sure you have some training in the induction period. Most packages have a 'play' mode to practise on.

Find out who the IT leads are in the practice, usually a member of practice staff and a GP. They will be the ones to turn to when the system crashes, the printers do not work or you have pressed the wrong button.

Establish the minimum computer-use expected of you. This will expand as the year progresses and by the end of your registrar year you should be familiar with day-to-day use, searches, making claims and using external links.

You may find it useful to attend specific courses on word-processing, data entry and presentation packages, particularly for the written work for summative assessment.

The computer in the consultation

Make sure you exit your last patient's notes before calling in the next one. Do not let your consultations be taken over by the computer.

Positioning your computer

Ideally your screen should be directly ahead of you. If this is not possible then the right-handed should have the computer on the right-hand side of the desk and the patient to the left (vice versa for left-handers). Do not have the computer as a barrier between you and the patient. You should have an adjustable chair so that your forearms are horizontal and your eyes the same height as the top of the screen. Have some space in front of the keyboard, or a wrist guard. Wrists should be kept straight. Neither you nor the screen should face windows or bright lights.

Data entry

Try to enter numbers as you take them e.g. weight, BMI and peak flow, even if you do most of your typing when the patient has left. With experience you will be able check medication, due-dates for smears and vaccinations and past history as you go. You should develop familiarity with frequently used 'Read codes' (see below).

If your practice uses both hand-written and computer records, ensure that some reference is made to the consultation in both.

Computer templates act as useful prompts, particularly for chronic diseases, health checks and contraception. Templates also make sure you enter information in codes consistent with other members of the practice, allowing for accurate audits.

Read codes

This coding system, in use throughout the NHS, allows clinical data to be entered according to a hierarchy system. As data is entered the computer software automatically offers you a choice of codes from fixed clinical labels. There may be more than one label for the same diagnosis so establish with your practice those most commonly used. This will help with future searches and audit.

Prescribing on the computer*

* See also Chapter 10: Prescribing.

- **Always check you are in the correct patient's file before prescribing.**
- **Check all the information on the printed prescription before signing it.**

Computers are extremely useful in prescribing:

- computer-generated scripts are legible and instantly recorded
- current and past medication easily traced
- generic equivalents easily found
- recorded allergies and significant interactions are flagged up.

You should be able to generate NHS or private prescriptions, prescribe for future issue and record anything issued by hand or a third party. A copy of the repeat medication list should be in the hand-held records. The right-hand section of the FP10 Comp can also be used to let the patient know about medication reviews, vaccination invitations and changes to practice details.

Links

Your practice may be electronically linked to:

* See GP income, p. 19.

- The *health authority* for item of service claims, obviating the need to fill out GMS forms.* Find out how this works and which practice staff member is responsible as you will be expected to make claims for contraception, minor surgery, etc.
- The *pathology/radiology service*, which speeds up the return of results. Clarify the practice policy for acting on and filing both the computer and paper results
- The *NHSnet*, which gives GPs direct access to hospital outpatient and day-case surgery appointments.

Databases

Systems usually have the scope for a practice phone directory. Find out how to use this to access, add and edit information on local NHS, private and voluntary sector services and contact numbers for practice doctors and staff.

Patient information leaflets may be available on a number of topics and can supplement other printed leaflets. The eBNF and medical decision support packages such as Prodigy or Mentor may also be available.

Audit, research and education

Use the computer for searches and organizing the data for your summative assessment written work. Classic medical texts such as the *Oxford Textbook of Medicine* are increasingly available on CD-ROM and the free trial CD is worth a look before you (or the practice) makes an investment. Many journals now have on-line formats, which you may be able to customize to your requirements.

Communications

Internal e-mail (intranet) is a useful way of circulating important practice and patient information, but can turn into yet another in-tray demanding your attention. The scope for connecting to the outside world is huge. Consider arranging some training at your VTS release course in using the internet to access peer-reviewed sites and to get the best out of Medline and the Cochrane database. Use our website address list[†] as a starting point.

† See Useful Addresses & Websites, p. 273.

Protecting patient information

The Data Protection Act (1998) governs the processing of information held in health, education and social services records, both manual and computerized. Processing includes obtaining, storing and disclosing information (*Box 11.3*).

Box 11.3   Selected Data Protection Principles (Data Protection Act 1998)

Data must be:
- relevant to the purpose for which it was obtained
- accurate
- kept up-to-date.

Appropriate security measures to protect data must be in place

Guidance is given on:
- sensitive information on race, ethnic origin, physical and mental health and sexual life
- material used for research purposes.

Practices must have a Data Protection Officer who is responsible for information handling and must register details and security measures with the Data Protection Commissioner. It is a criminal offence not to be registered under the act.

SOURCES AND FURTHER READING

1. Knight B. *Legal Aspects of Medical Practice*, 5th edn. Churchill Livingstone, 1992.
2. Lee N., Millman A. *ABC of Medical Computing*. BMJ Publishing Group, 1997.
3. Panting G., Lazarus R., Stearn M. *Medical Records*. Medical Protection Society, 1999.
4. GMC. *Confidentiality: Protecting and Providing Information*. GMC, 2000.
5. NHS Executive. *The Data Protection Act 1998. Protection and Use of Patient Information.* Health Service Circular HSC 2000/009, www.doh.gov.uk/coinh.htm
6. RCGP Information sheet no. 7. *General Practice Computerisation.* October 2000.
7. Health and Safety Executive. *Working with VDUs*, www.hse.gov.uk

12
Referrals

INTRODUCTION

GPs are obliged to arrange referrals for their patients to other services when necessary. With waiting times for outpatients and surgery continually in the public and political eye, we tread a fine line between serving our patients best without overloading secondary care.

Referral rates are increasing, reflecting a mixture of increased patient expectation, advances in medicine, poor social support and doctors' fear of litigation.

Individual GP referral patterns vary due to both patient and doctor factors, including difficulty tolerating uncertainty. Paradoxically, GPs with particular experience of a specialty may be more, not less, likely to refer to it.

You are responsible for the referrals you make and so must be confident of the qualifications of those you refer to. If you refer to non-medical practitioners then make sure they are members of a statutory regulatory body.

As a GP registrar you will refer a lot initially. You are expected to practise only within the limits of your expertise, so you should seek help if you are out of your depth. Don't opt for a best guess and don't worry about over-referring either. If all your referrals are appropriate you are probably not referring enough.

Invite consultants in the specialties in which you lack confidence to your VTS release course or ask if you can sit in on their out-patient clinics.*

* See also specialist hospital outpatients, p. 189.

This chapter looks at how best to refer your patients to secondary care and other services.

WHERE TO REFER

Spend a tutorial with your trainer working out how to refer patients to frequently used local services (*Box 12.1*).
Use information sources:

- trainer, GP colleagues and secretary
- local hospital handbook or directory of services
- local and national referral guidelines
- local hospital circulars on waiting times.

Build your own collected database of NHS, voluntary, complementary, private and self-help services.

Box 12.1   Directing your referrals

Identify:

Services offered within the practice and alternatives outside the practice:
- emergency IUCD insertions
- joint injections
- minor surgery
- drug dependency services.

Age cut-off for services for:
- paediatrics
- adolescents
- adults
- care of the elderly.

Gestation cut-off for gynaecology vs. obstetrics (usually 20 weeks)

Specialties accepting 'grey area' diagnoses such as:
- GI bleeds in the elderly
- pyelonephritis
- back pain.

Referral criteria for tertiary services:
- fertility
- plastic surgery.

Sexual health and reproductive medicine services:
- family planning
- termination of pregnancy
- early pregnancy unit
- genitourinary medicine.

One-stop diagnostic clinics e.g:
- haematuria
- post-menopausal bleeding
- pigmented lesions.

Paediatric walk-in clinics

Talking therapy services:
- counselling
- cognitive behavioural therapy
- psycho-sexual counselling
- psychotherapy.

EMERGENCY REFERRALS

In or out-of-hours, arranging urgent hospital assessment or admission is time-consuming and can be particularly disruptive mid-surgery. Enlist the help of your practice staff for administrative tasks (bleeping the on-call doctors or arranging an ambulance). Some hospitals have a centralized system or a nursing manager to accept calls for emergency GP referrals, during working hours.

Getting your patient accepted

Speak to the on call team. If the problem is not straightforward, as with many GP referrals, and you are likely to have to 'sell' the case, spend a few moments collecting your thoughts and clinical findings before you contact the hospital team. You are more likely to get your patient seen with a minimum of fuss if you ask for an *assessment*, rather than an *admission*. You may be more experienced than many of the SHOs so do not allow yourself to be bullied. You only need to have done a clinical assessment sufficient to ascertain whether the patient requires referral. You do not need to do a rectal or vaginal examination unless it would change your diagnosis or management. It is unfair to put the patient through an unpleasant examination that will inevitably be repeated.

In the few situations where the on-call doctor refuses a referral, without good reason and an alternative management plan, you can advise them that you will need to discuss the case with their consultant. This is rarely needed, but the consultant will invariably accept the patient on behalf of their team.

Sending the patient in

Send a hand-written referral letter with the patient or fax a letter to A&E for the attention of the admitting team. Ensure you keep a copy for the medical record. Give the patient clear instructions as to where they are to go, which team is expecting them and whether they can expect to be admitted. Do not attempt a guess at how soon they will be seen, but explain that they will be seen more quickly than the 'minor injuries' because they have been referred directly to a specialist team. You may find patients reluctant to be referred for possible admission so you may have to be persuasive (see below).

Arranging an ambulance

If the patient is seriously ill or has no safe way of travelling to hospital then arrange an ambulance (*Box 12.2*).

*Reproduced from *Information for GPs and Clinicians* (London Ambulance Service) March 1998.

Keep a record of the GP priority ambulance phone number in your medical bag; otherwise call 999. Give reception staff full patient details for ambulance control (*Box 12.2*) if you delegate this task to them. You will be given a reference number, which should be documented in the patient's medical record together with the time of the request, so delays can be chased up.

In some conditions, for example asthma, it may be safer for the patient to wait for an ambulance than to be taken in their own car and you should stay with the patient until the ambulance arrives.

If it is clear from a phone consultation that a 999 ambulance is needed, arrange this and try to get to the patient yourself if you can. If you do not make it before the ambulance then inform A&E or the specialist team of the patient's impending arrival.

Patients refusing emergency referral

Some patients will refuse urgent referral when you consider it imperative. Explain to them you are referring them for an assessment and that they can later refuse admission if it is offered. Ask yourself:

See The Mental Health Act and the acutely mentally ill patient, p. 250.

† See Competence (the capacity to make decisions), p. 226.

‡ See Treating incompetent adults: 'best interests' principle, p. 227.

- Is the patient mentally ill and a danger to themselves or others? If so, a mental health section may be required.* Only mental illness and physical illness arising from that mental illness can be treated under the Mental Health Act, not physical illness alone
- Is the patient competent to decide for themselves?† If they are not competent, for example in an acute confusional state, you may act in their best interests and refer, but be prepared to justify this.‡ Restraint and tranquillizing drugs may be used. You should be protected under common law (against an accusation of assault) in such situations.

If the patient *is* competent then you cannot force them to accept referral for admission. Try to find out why they are refusing, for example hospital phobia, death of their spouse in hospital or fear of long A&E wait, and address their fears. You have a duty to explain why you feel it necessary to refer them and make clear the possible consequences of their refusal. Be honest about the possible outcomes of their refusal but do not scaremonger. If they still refuse then respect their decision, document it fully in the notes and arrange the best alternative care (*Box 12.3*).

Box 12.3 Alternatives to admission

- Symptomatic treatment and a planned review
- An urgent (same week) outpatient appointment
- Day hospital assessment (care of elderly, psychiatric)
- Domiciliary visit by specialist (liaison psychiatry team, psychogeriatrician)
- Referral to the palliative care team

Private emergency referrals

Although some private hospitals have a centralized admission system for urgent referrals, these can be difficult to arrange as you may need to contact a willing private specialist, hospital and private ambulance service yourself. Encourage patients in emergency situations to use an NHS facility. Reassure them that true emergencies are handled quickly by the NHS and that private hospitals may be less well-equipped to deal with some emergencies. Patients can always negotiate a private transfer with their consultant once they are over the acute stage.

NON-EMERGENCY REFERRALS

Referrals to Primary Health Care Team colleagues and social services

Referrals to district nurses, health visitors or social services can be done in person, over the phone or via a referral book, but should always be afforded the same respect as other referrals. Make clear the reason for your referral and state exactly what you want from the service, (for example continence assessment, ulcer dressing or just 'assessment'). You should receive feedback in practice meetings with members of the PHCT.

Outpatient referrals*

* See also Arranging NHS terminations, p. 258.

These will form the bulk of your referrals. Check if the patient has a preference as to where or to whom they are referred within the confines of your local contracts. Letters addressed to 'Dear colleague' are usually passed to the consultant with the shortest wait in the specialty.

Discuss cases that require urgent outpatient assessment with the specialist registrar or even consultant and then fax, as well as send, your referral letter reiterating the urgency of the case.

It is useful to discuss some less urgent cases with the relevant team, particularly unclear problems. This may obviate the need for referral or allow you to start treatment before the appointment.

Tell the patient the specialty to which they have been referred (and explain what an endocrinologist or a urologist is). Be honest about how long they are likely to wait for their appointment, give them an idea of when they should hear from the hospital and a contact number for them to chase up their appointment if necessary. Unfortunately lost referrals and appointment cancellations are a common occurrence in the current inefficient system. Delegate chasing-up appointments to your practice staff.

Make it clear to patients that they should come back to you should their symptoms change or deteriorate. You can expedite their appointment, in which case you may need to speak to the specialist team directly. Similarly ask those who have improved and no longer need a specialist opinion to cancel their appointments.

Referrals to professions allied to medicine

Physiotherapy, occupational therapy, midwifery and talking therapies may be offered as hospital and community services. They often have forms and specific guidelines for referrals. You may wish to speak to them individually, particularly for complex or urgent cases.

Private referrals

Use recommendations from your trainer, consultants you have worked with and the local NHS hospital specialists who work privately. Find out who provides local private physiotherapy, osteopathy and radiology services.

In contrast to NHS appointments, patients usually contact the specialists' secretary directly to arrange their appointment. Give them the specialist's contact details and leave a referral letter for them to collect and take to the appointment.

Those with private health insurance should contact their insurance company for prior agreement for the referral and a claim form. Forewarn them that the practice charges a fee for completion of such forms.

If you feel a private specialist opinion is not justified for a problem that can be managed in general practice then it is acceptable not to refer but explain why. If the patient is not happy with this then suggest they discuss it with one of the partners.

Those who wish to pay their own way do not need your 'blessing'. Strictly speaking they do not need a referral letter either, although it is good practice to write one.

Discuss any problems that arise with private insurance claim forms with your trainer.

Complementary therapy referrals

With the increasing popularity and acknowledged effectiveness of some of these therapies, GPs are increasingly expected to advise and refer. Although there are some NHS osteopathy and acupuncture services, most still require the patient to pay. If you do not know what the therapy involves or doubt its effectiveness then say so. You may provide patients with contact details so they can do their own research, but make it clear you are not formally recommending the treatment or referring them. Osteopaths and chiropractors have their own regulatory body, and it is reasonable to rely on membership of these as evidence of training.

Invite complementary practitioners to talk at your VTS release course to inform you on their therapies.

REFERRAL LETTERS

> **Make clear to your secretary the priority of all your referrals:**
> * **emergency – same day**
> * **urgent – within a few days**
> * **routine – anything longer.**

> **Patients with a possible diagnosis of cancer should be referred the same day and see a specialist within 2 weeks.**

Reduce your paperwork by identifying the services that allow self-referral, for example social services, drug dependency and podiatry for elderly, and use referral proformas where available.

Aim to do all your letters after each surgery while the problem is fresh in your mind. Otherwise ensure you have marked each set of notes clearly with a 'Post-it' note with the required action and catch up weekly.

Your practice should provide you with a 'dictaphone' and you should keep a spare tape in your room. Be kind to your secretary/typist (*Box 12.4*).

Dictation is usually quickest (although some GPs will write by hand or even type themselves) and takes practice, so use our guide initially (*Box 12.5*). Your referral letters will be seen by many people, including the patient, so do yourself justice.

Correct typing errors and aim to sign all your own letters before they go out. Signing outgoing letters for absent partners can reveal different styles, problems and consultant preferences. Overall practice referral

Box 12.4   Dictation tips

- Start the tape with an introduction such as 'Dr X's' letters on Tuesday 4th May'
- Dictate urgent letters on a separate tape or first on the tape
- Speak clearly and slowly
- Spell difficult medical and other long words
- Give clear grammatical directions: 'Full stop. New paragraph'
- Make the addressee clear: 'Dear Dr' or a specific consultant
- Stipulate:
  - NHS or private
  - urgent or routine
  - for faxing, sending or collection by patient
  - whether a fee will be incurred (to be marked on the envelope).
- Give clear instructions on enclosures such as copies of results/ old letters/invoices
- Request that important words are highlighted or in bold (**'URGENT'**, **'? Rectal carcinoma'**)
- Do not put too many letters on one tape
- Affix tape securely to notes, or put in an envelope marked with the patients' names

Box 12.5   Referral letters: essential contents

- Consultants prioritize most outpatient appointments on the basis of your letter
- Be concise but complete
- Ensure a copy is kept in the medical record.
- Include:
    - Full patient details and current phone number – confirm these with patient
    - NHS number and hospital number if known
    - Patient's problem as a title before the text, for example, 'Right Inguinal Hernia'
    - Brief and relevant history
    - Any treatment tried to date
    - Any investigations to date (with copies of results)
    - Reason for the referral, for example:
        hospital involvement essential
        second opinion (at your or the patient's request)
        exclusion of a serious diagnosis
        diagnostic uncertainty
        treatment failure.
- List only relevant and significant past medical and family history
- List current regular medication
- List known allergies
- State what you have told the patient in cases of a potentially serious diagnosis, for example 'I have explained to the patient that MS is a possible diagnosis'
- Request transport and translators if needed

data may be available on the computer. Spend a tutorial reviewing your own referrals for a week to reflect on their appropriateness and style.

SOURCES AND FURTHER READING

1. GMC. *Good Medical Practice.* GMC, July 1998.
2. GMC. *Seeking patients' consent: the ethical considerations.* GMC, November 1998.
3. NICE. *Referral Cues Project,* April 2000, www.nice.org.uk
4. National Association of Non-Principals. *Standardised Practice Induction Pack.*
5. London Ambulance Service NHS Trust. *Information for GPs and Clinicians.* LAS, March 1998.

13
Investigations and results

INTRODUCTION

Organizing investigations and dealing with results involves a lot of work and can throw up many decision-making dilemmas. Tests are also costly to the NHS.

Remember:

* See Understanding consent, p. 224.

- You should always have a patient's informed consent before undertaking any investigation. Whilst this is generally implied by the patient's attendance (such as for a blood test), you should always confirm it. You may need explicit consent for some investigations such as HIV tests*
- The practice should have a fail-safe system for processing all results
- Follow-up of all abnormal results is essential and the responsibility of the requesting doctor.

WHERE TO ORGANIZE YOUR TESTS

Find out from your trainer where most of the common GP investigations are carried out (*Box 13.1*). Local hospitals should have direct access for GP patients for basic investigations, often without appointment and at times specified on the request forms. Other investigations may require specialist referral.

Box 13.1 Hospital investigation services for GP patients

Confirm local availability
- Phlebotomy
- Paediatric:
  - phlebotomy
  - bag urine sample.
- Simple radiology/ultrasound
- Specialist radiology (barium studies, venogram, IVP)
- ECG
- Echocardiography
- Exercise ECG
- Endoscopy
- *H. pylori* breath testing
- Bone density scanning

WHICH TESTS

Generally speaking, GP investigations will be for diagnostic, screening or monitoring purposes, although they can also be used, with discretion, to buy time when you are unsure how to manage an unclear presentation.* Be wary of over-investigating. This can increase patient expectations and may be actively unhelpful by colluding with somatizing patients. Limit all your investigations to the simple ones that will help your management. Avoid 'serum rhubarbs'.

* See What to do when you don't know what to do, p. 88.

Most investigations will be:

- near-patient tests – peak flow, BM stix, urinalysis, pregnancy tests (in which case do not forget to document the results)
- laboratory tests – basic bloods, MSUs, stools, swabs and cervical smears
- X-rays and ultrasound.

Nursing staff also generate investigations and you will need to act upon these results too.

Monitoring chronic conditions and drug treatment

There is often little consensus over the exact frequency of investigations and review for chronic diseases or drug monitoring so be guided by your colleagues and hospital specialists. Computer prompts and diary due-dates can help ensure patients are followed up. These areas lend themselves nicely to audit.

Check opportunistically in consultations if repeat tests are required, otherwise leave messages and pathology request forms with repeat prescriptions.

As with prescribing, clarify and document clearly who is responsible for arranging tests for those patients under shared specialist and GP care.† Update the medical record with relevant test results from hospital letters.‡

† See also Patients under shared hospital and GP care, p. 101.

‡ See also Clinical post, p. 158.

Screening tests

Screening is an important part of general practice, and a big topic for the MRCGP exam.

Given the uncertainties involved in some screening tests and the potentially serious consequences of a positive test, you must be sufficiently informed to counsel patients adequately (*Box 13.2*). Have a tutorial or VTS meeting on the subject.

Explain

- The purpose of the screening
- The likelihood of false positives and negatives
- The uncertainties and risks involved in the process
- Significant medical, social or financial implications of the screening
- Follow-up plans

Ensure your patients know how and when they should receive the results of any screening test. Your practice should have a fail-safe system for processing cervical smear results, so find out how this works. Breast screening is usually organized by the health authority, but the GP has an important role in reinforcing its importance.

Antenatal screening tests

Screening in pregnancy can generate enormous anxiety and raise many difficult questions. Clarify exactly:

- what tests are offered to women at your local antenatal service
- who (GP or midwives) is responsible for chasing up the basic antenatal screening tests and
- how the woman can access her results.

If you are responsible for organizing the tests make sure you are well-informed and allow enough time to discuss these in early antenatal appointments. Use written information on the statistics of risk, and of procedures such as amniocentesis, to back up your discussions where possible. Give the woman and her partner an opportunity to ask questions.*

* See also Breaking bad news, p. 89.

ORGANIZING TESTS

Document fully all investigations you organize in the medical record.

Lost or unlabelled specimens generate unnecessary work for you and inconvenience for your patient so take care when dealing with specimens (*Box 13.3*).

Box 13.3   Processing specimens

- Adhere to local practice policy on sharps and infection control when dealing with all specimens
- Label all specimen pots/carriers with full name, date of birth and date sample taken
- Ensure lids are secured and plastic transport bags well sealed (with staples or sticky tape if necessary)
- Complete pathology form legibly and fully and add your personal 'labcode' so results are directed back to you
- Identify:
  - outgoing sample basket
  - overnight storage fridge (cervical smears and some swabs do not need refrigeration).
- Advise patients of specimen collection times from the surgery (and that they can drop samples to pathology themselves)
- Document all investigations arranged in the medical record
- Share responsibility with the patient for following up their results

---

Delegate phlebotomy to hospital phlebotomists or your practice nurse, unless you are on a home visit or with an acutely ill patient.

Practices should keep a record of all specimens sent from the practice to check that all results are received. This is usually in place for cervical smears at least, and may be the job of the practice nurse or reception staff.

Keep a personal record of particularly important tests you request so you can follow them up yourself. In every case you should pass some responsibility for accessing the results back to the patient, or carer. Explain the system for doing so, ensure they know exactly how many test results to expect and give them a realistic time-frame.

If you agree to arrange investigations in a phone encounter, then leave completed pathology forms at reception for collection.

Urgent requests

Pathology

Check local protocols. In general you should phone ahead to the relevant laboratory or bleep the duty technician. Ask for the results to be phoned or faxed back the same day. Mark the request form 'urgent' and ensure practice contact details are clear. You may need to organize special transport for the specimen. Make arrangements with the duty doctor to chase up results later if you will not be available yourself.

Radiology

Phone the department directly. Same-day gynaecology ultrasound scans to exclude ectopic pregnancy can often be accommodated easily. Other imaging may require specific discussion with the on-call radiologist. You may need to fax the request form.

Housebound patients

On routine home visits take any necessary bloods yourself, otherwise ask the practice or district nurse. If an elderly patient needs several investigations as well, such as an ECG and CXR, then consider referring them to the day hospital for a full work-up for which transport can be arranged.

Uncommon tests

Check with the pathology laboratory the bottle or container required for unusual or unfamiliar tests you request. Make this clear on the request form for your practice nurse or phlebotomist if you are not taking the sample yourself.

Some tests may only be undertaken at particular times (semen samples) or by specialist centres (genetic screening), so contact the relevant laboratory for more information.

You will occasionally be asked to take bloods for a patient as part of a research project or for a private medical. The kit will usually be supplied and you will need to send it back in the post. Check if there is a fee payable.

Patients may request tests that are unusual in daily general practice, such as selenium levels or 'allergy tests', or have been recommended by a complementary practitioner. These situations can be difficult to manage. Try to discover any underlying worries that may reveal a simpler problem. Talk it through with your trainer, or hospital laboratory and consider a specialist referral if necessary. Do not arrange investigations if you will not be able to interpret the results.

Beware the patient who seems to want 'testing for everything'. There is usually an underlying agenda, which you will need to unravel sensitively.

Patients refusing tests

Patients sometimes opt out of investigations, preferring to wait and see, or decide not to have them done simply because they get better. Difficulties arise when patients actively refuse investigations that you consider clinically important. Approach these situations as you would patients refusing referral.* Ask them why they are declining (dislike of needles can be overcome by using local anaesthetic cream or talking therapies). Explain fully your reasons for requesting the investigation and the consequences of not having it.

See Patients refusing emergency referral, p. 129.

If you feel they are competent to refuse† then respect their wishes, document your explanation and their refusal in the medical record and arrange alternative management.

† See Refusal of consent, p. 227.

Difficult situations include the elderly confused patient who may have a treatable cause for their mental state and those with severe learning disabilities whom you suspect have a physical problem yet are unable to cooperate. Discuss such dilemmas with your trainer.

Private tests

Ask your trainer for details of a local private pathology and radiology service for the occasional patient who will not want to wait for the NHS service. Ensure you complete forms (or request letters) fully with your personal and practice details so results are returned appropriately.

DEALING WITH RESULTS

> *It is your responsibility to ensure that you have seen and acted on results of all the tests you request.*

Your practice will have a system for processing all incoming results (both paper and electronic versions) and for patients to access their results.

Paper results should be date-stamped and directed to the requesting doctor. They may also be stamped with a variety of options for your action (*Box 13.4.*)

Box 13.4   Practice results stamp instructions

- Seen by Dr ...
- Tell patient normal
- File
- Pull notes for Dr ...
- Ask patient to phone Dr ...
- Ask patient to make appointment
- Needs repeat, form left for collection
- Ask patient to collect prescription
- Other

* See also Clinical post, p. 158.

† See Ensuring paperwork is viewed in your absence, p. 158.

Sign or initial all your results.* If you are away then ensure that someone sees your results in your absence.†

Some practices document all results in a book which is used to relay results and action to patients when they enquire. Receptionists must give out only the doctor's instructions and not specific clinical information. Written notification of all cervical smear results (normal or not) should be sent to the woman.

Results taken over the phone should be documented in the medical record and marked as such ('T') in case errors occurred in transcribing. Make sure you also see the paper version.

Ask reception staff to chase up any results not available in the medical record which you need mid-surgery.

Always include copies of relevant test results in your outpatient referral letters.

Linked results

If your practice is electronically linked to the local laboratory results may be filed directly in the patient's computer medical record. Paper results will arrive later so the practice should have a clear policy for dealing with both to ensure results are acted on without duplicating work.

Abnormal results

Straightforward

Simple abnormal results such as confirmed UTI or positive throat swab should be easy to deal with:

- check current treatment in the medical record
- if treatment is needed contact the patient by phone or letter depending on urgency (you may be able to delegate this to nursing or reception staff)
- arrange appropriate management (such as prescriptions, further investigations and leave forms at reception)
- document your actions in the medical record and on the report itself.

Patients should be invited in for an appointment for abnormal screening tests that may have significant implications such as haemoglobinopathies or markedly elevated cholesterol levels.

The laboratory may add a helpful interpretation or suggest an action such as 'Notify'‡ or suggest rubella vaccination.

‡ See Notifiable diseases, p. 256.

Seriously abnormal results

Dangerously abnormal results (high INR or elevated potassium) and less acute, but serious abnormalities (possible lung cancer) will usually be phoned through to you. Contact the patient with a management plan, which may include urgent hospital referral or arrangements for a repeat test or an urgent consultation.*

* See also Breaking bad news, p. 89.

Mildly abnormal or 'unclear' results

These can present problems, particularly if you are dealing with results of a patient you do not know well. Review the medical records and use your clinical judgement. Arrange a repeat test if necessary to see the trend of the abnormality and ask for advice from your GP or specialist colleagues. Sometimes it is appropriate to ignore the result and reassure the patient it is not clinically significant.

SOURCES AND FURTHER READING

1. GMC, *Seeking patients' consent: the ethical considerations.* GMC, November 1998.
2. UK National Screening Committee, www.doh.gov.uk/nsc/index.htm

14
Statutory medical certificates and benefits

INTRODUCTION

GPs are obliged to issue statutory certificates for patients unable to work due to ill-health. Sick certificates (also referred to as 'sick lines' by some patients) entitle the employed to claim Statutory Sick Pay, and the unemployed to claim state incapacity benefits. State benefits are administered by the Department for Work and Pensions (DWP). Certification can present problems for the GP who has a responsibility to both the patient and the DWP. The DWP produces a useful guide for doctors on completing certificates; *Publication IB204, A Guide for Registered Medical Practitioners* also available on-line.

Patients also request certificates for a wide variety of other reasons, completion of which is not necessarily part of a GP's NHS work.*

The benefits system is complex and ever-changing. Few GPs have a full grasp of the benefits and allowances for which their patients are eligible. It is highly satisfying to advise a patient on a benefit to which they did not know they were entitled.

This chapter covers issues relating to England, Wales and Scotland. Northern Ireland may have slight differences in forms and agencies to those discussed here.

* See Form- filling, letter-writing and other certificates, p. 158.

SICKNESS CERTIFICATES

There are several statutory certificates available with differing stipulations (*Box 14.1*). You should familiarize yourself with them and their accurate completion (*Box 14.2*). Document the details of any

---

Box 14.1   Which statutory medical certificate?

None	1–3 days illness
Self-certificate (SC1 or 2)	3–7 days illness
Med 3	After 7 days illness
	Open: no fixed return date
	Closed: return date stated within 14 days
Med 5	Backdated – on basis of previous consultation or report from another doctor, for example discharge summary within last month
Med 4	Requested prior to Personal Capability Assessment (PCA)

Reproduced from *IB204: A guide for registered medical practitioners*, Department of Work and Pensions.

certificate you issue (e.g. Med 3, flu-like illness, 1 week) in the medical record.

Self-certificates

Usually no statutory certificate is needed for absences of up to 3 working days. For absences between 3 and 7 days patients can complete a self-certificate (SC1 for the unemployed and SC2 for employed patients), which are available from employers, the surgery or post offices. Employers should accept an SC2 and not expect GPs to issue certificates for short absences (see Private sick notes below). With an SC1 certificate, those on Job Seeker's Allowance are entitled to benefit without having to be actively looking for work for a short period.

Med 3

A statement of incapacity to work, the Med 3, must be issued on the day of the consultation or within 24 hours. It can be 'open' with no specific return date, for example 4 weeks, or 'closed' when a specific return to work date is agreed within the next 14 days. Within the first 6 months of illness a certificate can only be issued for up to 6 months. After this any time can be stipulated, even 'indefinite'.

Med 5

A special statement of incapacity to work, the Med 5, is issued under the following circumstances:

- Backdated, when a doctor agrees to issue a certificate based on their examination on a previous occasion to cover a period in the past. In these circumstances a Med 3 cannot be issued as over 24 hours have elapsed since the patient was seen. The doctor must be sure that they would have advised the patient to refrain from work for the entire period of the certificate. It can also be used to sign the patient off work for a further period of up to 4 weeks
- On the basis of a report from another doctor, for example after an in-patient stay when you are in receipt of the discharge summary. The report must not be more than a month old.

You *cannot* issue a Med 5 if you have not seen the patient during the period of illness or have not received a report from another doctor who has seen the patient.

Med 4

A patient claiming a state incapacity benefit may be asked to undergo a Personal Capability Assessment (PCA, see below). The PCA is usually applied after 28 weeks of incapacity but, depending on the medical condition, may be applied much earlier than this. The patient will be sent a questionnaire to complete themselves and asked to obtain a Med 4 from their doctor. The completion of the Med 4 over-rides any previous Med 3 certificates and should be completed with particular care to include:

- main diagnosis for incapacity
- any other illnesses
- effect of illness on function and ability to perform usual occupation
- treatment and prognosis
- ability of the patient to travel up to 90 minutes for the PCA.

Certain conditions will exempt a patient from attending for a PCA, for example tetraplegia or registered blindness, so careful completion may help your patient avoid an unnecessary examination.

Med 6

Very occasionally doctors judge it not to be in their patient's best interests to put a true or accurate diagnosis, for example malignancy, on a Med 3, 4 or 5. In these circumstances a Med 6, found at the back of the Med 3 and Med 4 pads, should be completed and sent to the local benefits office (address in the telephone directory). A fuller medical report may then be requested.

RM7

On the rare occasion you would like a patient to have a PCA before 28 weeks, because you doubt their incapacity but have issued a certificate, then send an RM7 (found at the back of the Med 3 pad) to the local benefits office.

DS1500

The DS1500 form should be completed for patients with a potentially terminal illness, who are likely to die within the next 6 months. This entitles the patient to 'special rules' that enable them to receive the highest rate for Attendance Allowance (AA), Disability Living Allowance (DLA), or Incapacity Benefit. Check they have already made a claim for these. A fee is payable for completing the form.

Private sick notes

Patients often request certificates for less than 7 days absence for their employers. The national guidelines of certification have been carefully negotiated and GPs are not obliged to issue such certificates unless specifically requested by the DWP.

If a patient or employer insists on a certificate then a private sick certificate or note can be issued at your discretion and a fee can be charged. This may be hand-written or on a practice proforma. Include a minimum of information and remain mindful of protecting the patient's confidentiality. You may wish to add 'further details are available on request with the patient's permission'.

Practices may produce a leaflet for patients to give to their employer explaining the rules of certification. Employers can be asked to write to the GP to confirm the patient's attendance.

Difficulties arise where patients request letters for illness episodes for which they have not consulted a doctor. If you do agree to such requests then state that 'this patient *informs* me that they have been unwell' as you cannot actually confirm their illness.

FITNESS TO WORK

There are no absolute stipulations on the amount of time off work required for specific conditions although the DWP is developing some evidence-based guidance. Hospital specialists should give advice after an inpatient stay or operation and should issue the initial certificate.

There are great individual variations in recovery times and psychological issues can prolong recovery. Depression, dislike of a job or boss and high local levels of unemployment can be contributing factors. A prolonged absence from work may not be in the best interests of some patients so try to avoid colluding with them. Use your judgement, backed up with clinical evidence, for example back pain guidelines, to decide what is in the patient's best interest regarding their fitness to work. If you suspect depression is an underlying issue then address this. Conversely persuading some patients that they need time off can be a problem, particularly if they are self-employed.

Early advice and encouragement from a GP can enable some patients to get back to work and prevent the poverty and social isolation associated with long-term incapacity.

Negotiating sickness certificates: difficult cases

It is acceptable to sign people off work with a largely psychological condition such as stress, to allow them a short period of recovery time when they are overwhelmed by stressors or life crises, rather than illness.

Difficult situations arise where a patient requests a sickness certificate, yet you feel it is inappropriate. Take time to explore the patient's agenda and to explain your reasons if you still consider it inappropriate. If problems at work are a contributing factor, then encourage the patient to discuss these with their employer. Sometimes you can negotiate and agree to sign them off until a certain date, after which they should be reviewed and strongly encouraged to return to work. Discuss difficult cases with your trainer or the GP the patient usually sees.

Personal Capability Assessment (PCA)

This clinical examination is undertaken by independent doctors, 'approved' by the DWP, to ascertain a long-term claimant's fitness to do any sort of work, not necessarily their own job.

A person is asked to undergo a PCA usually after a period of incapacity of 6 months. The level of assessment is based on the person's ability to perform certain day-to-day functions, and if reduced to a certain point they may be entitled to benefit without being expected to seek work.

The GP who has been issuing the patient with sick notes may be sent an IB113 form for completion before the PCA takes place, which requests detailed information on the patient's current illness, treatment and prognosis.

Once a PCA had been 'applied' (or passed), and the patient deemed unfit for work, their GP will be informed and further certificates will not be needed during that spell of incapacity.

Working with disability

It is reasonable to write to employers in support of reduced duties for those who have been off work for serious illness or injury for some time and are slowly integrating themselves back into work. These details can also be included on a closed Med 3.

The Disability Discrimination Act (1995) requires employers to make reasonable adjustments to the workplace for employees with long-term disability.

Disability Employment Advisors and Disability Service Teams should provide such individuals with advice and support on staying in employment, returning to work and starting work after a long absence.

As well as 'incapacity' benefits there are also 'in work' benefits making work a financially advantageous option.

MATERNITY CERTIFICATES

Mat B1

Issued by a doctor or midwife within 20 weeks of the expected week of confinement, (i.e. at 20 weeks gestation), the Mat B1 allows women to claim Statutory Maternity Pay (SMP) if employed or Maternity Allowance (MA) if not. Both are paid up to a maximum of 18 weeks, starting 11 weeks before the expected week of confinement at the earliest.

If a woman is not entitled to SMP or MA (usually because not enough National Insurance has been paid), she may be treated as incapable of work from 6 weeks before expected delivery to 14 weeks after and issued a Med 3.

Sure Start Maternity Grant

Sure Start Maternity Grant (SSMG) is payable to low-income families to help with the costs of a new baby. Parents must have received advice from a medical professional on maternal and child health-care issues and have a signed form from a doctor or midwife to confirm this before making a claim.

BENEFITS

Millions of pounds a year are lost to patients in unclaimed benefits. Increased income from benefits (*Box 14.3*) can positively improve the health of individuals. Entitlement to some benefits depends on previous National Insurance contributions.

GPs have an obligation to complete forms used for assessing eligibility for benefits. As a GP registrar you will not be expected to complete many of these, but patients will ask you for advice and it is salutary to go through the occasional one to see the work involved.

Box 14.3 Main DWP benefits 2001

Benefit	Eligibility
Incapacity Benefit	• Payable if unable to work through illness or disability.
	• Med 3 issued by GP until PCA applied.
Income Support	• Tops up income for low-income households where people are not expected to be looking for work.
	• Carers, single parents, elderly and those unable to work full-time because of illness are eligible.
	• Entitles claimants to other benefits, e.g. housing, council tax and health costs.
Disabled Person's Tax Credit (DPTC)	• For those working but restricted in type or hours of work due to illness or disability.
Disability Living Allowance (DLA)	• Under-65s.
	• Disabled and need either care or supervision or have reduced mobility.
	• Two components: mobility and care.
	• Higher and lower rates depend on level of disability and care needed.
Attendance Allowance (AA)	• Over-65s needing care and/or supervision from another person.
Blue Badge (previously orange)	• Parking concessions for the disabled and their drivers.
	• Application to social services.

Keep up-to-date with the basics. Good information sources include:

- DWP website www.dwp.gov.uk
- Citizens' Advice Bureau (keep the number handy in your surgery)
- benefits advice workers who may be attached to your surgery or community centres
- the *Oxford Handbook of Patients' Welfare*, an excellent guide for doctors, which also has on-line updates
- the GP press, which periodically publishes 'cut out and keep' guides to benefit, voluntary and self-help organizations.

SOURCES AND FURTHER READING

1. Sandell A. *Oxford Handbook of Patients' Welfare*. Oxford University Press, 1998.
2. Department for Work and Pensions. *Publication IB204; a Guide for Registered Medical Practitioners*, April 2000, available from DWP website, www.dwp.gov.uk
3. Citizens' Advice Bureau website, www.nacab.org.uk
4. NHS A to Z Help-direct website, www.nhsatoz.org

15
Paperwork

INTRODUCTION

The volume of GP paperwork has increased dramatically over the last decade due to increased NHS bureaucracy and patient and third-party demands, some of which can seem ridiculous. Fortunately there is currently a government initiative to cut GP involvement in unnecessary paperwork, particularly the non-clinical elements.

Although as a GP registrar you will have nothing like the volume of a partner's paperwork, developing good habits for dealing with it will stand you in good stead in the future. You may be expected to go through absent partners' post and this can be an eye-opener as to what they have to contend with on a daily basis (*Box 15.1*).

Box 15.1 Making sense of incoming mail

Patient-related
- Pathology and radiology results
- Hospital letters
- Private specialist letters
- Communications from patients (including prescriptions and referral requests)
- Statutory and private forms for completion for third parties
- Requests for letters, e.g.'fitness to …' certificates

NHS-related communications from:
- Chief Medical Officer
- Department of Health
- NHS Executive
- Health authority/PCG/PCT
- National guidelines.

Political information from:
- BMA
- GPC
- LMC.

Education and training
- Notifications of meetings
- Training updates/courses

Journals
- Including the GP press: *Pulse, GP, Doctor.*

Promotional material from:
- drug companies
- private hospitals consultants
- medical equipment suppliers.

Other
- Questionnaires
- Teaching/research

Practice administration
- Should be directed to the practice manager

DEALING WITH PAPERWORK

All incoming mail should be opened by clerical staff, date-stamped and directed to the individual GP's in-tray. In an ideal world forms should land in your in-tray with basic details already completed by the patient and with the medical records attached.

Organizing yourself

Deal with the paperwork arising from consultations after each surgery together with your phone messages and e-mails and go through your incoming post daily. Aim to clear your in-tray daily, although this may be difficult on on-call days. Use the midday gap between surgeries to process paperwork and set aside a weekly slot to catch up with the more time-consuming tasks (and to follow up patients causing you concern). Make use of surgery time when patients fail to turn up, but be sensible about what you can manage in the time available; do not start a complicated report or letter if you only have 7 minutes.

Some GPs prefer to use early mornings for paperwork when they are fresh and there are fewer interruptions. As a GP registrar you should never need to take patient-related work home with you.

If you also receive medical mail at home then set aside a specific time to deal with it. Blitz your accumulated paperwork every month or two and dispose of anything irrelevant or out of date.

Time-saving measures

- Prioritize the clinically relevant post and organize the rest in your 'to do' basket (*Box 15.2*). Ideally you should handle, and deal with, each piece of paper only once
- Delegate. Redirect items to other GPs if they know the patient well and expect them to do the same to you. Use administrative staff to fax, call patients and chase results and appointments
- Contact the medical mailing lists (usually found at the back of the GP publications) to cancel subscriptions if you are inundated with unsolicited mail at home or work

---

Box 15.2   Prioritizing paperwork

- Urgent   Do it now, certainly today
- Soon   This week
- File   Future reference
- 'Bumph'   Bin

Clinical post

Sign or initial everything you deal with, even if normal, and make clear any action undertaken. Put the 'normals' into filing and the others in a file marked 'Pull notes for Dr X'. Give this to a member of staff and catch up with the notes later in your in-tray.

Update patients' medical and prescribing records with significant results, new diagnoses, and drug changes instituted in hospital. Some practices employ a staff member to upload the computer with relevant data you have highlighted on letters.

If you are unsure of what, or whether, action is required then discuss it with your trainer. Hospital letters can sometimes be rather ambiguous, for example who is responsible for prescribing for a patient,* so you may need to contact the hospital. Similarly, seek advice if you are dealing with an absent partner's post and unsure whether or not to act now or leave it until the partner's return.

* See also Patients under shared hospital and GP care, p. 101.

Ensuring paperwork is viewed in your absence

Ask a GP colleague to go through your post and act on urgent matters while you are away. They should leave significant items and the action taken in your in-tray for you to see on your return.

You may also need to arrange with your practice manager to have an hour or two of surgery time blocked out for you to catch up with your post in your first surgery back.

Educational material, circulars and journals

Avoid building up a depressing 'journal-mountain' (*Box 15.3*). Use coffee breaks and slots when patients fail to attend for the lighter reading and set aside a weekly time to read those items that need more brain engagement. Extract and keep relevant information in your developing filing system for clinical reference and the exams.

FORM-FILLING, LETTER-WRITING AND OTHER CERTIFICATES

* See Chapter 14: Statutory medical certificates and benefits.

Aside from requests for sick notes* GPs receive numerous requests for forms and letters on behalf of their patients. Some of these are fairly loosely related to medicine, for example fitness to be in the school play. GPs are not necessarily obliged to fulfil some of these requests and may actively refuse. Hopefully the obligation to complete some of these will be removed in the government's GP paperwork-reduction initiative.

> **Box 15.3 Keeping on top of the medical journals**
>
> - Identify and limit yourself to the few you really need (see Chapter 21: The MRCGP Exam, and 'hot topics', and discuss with your trainer and VTS colleagues)
> - Reduce your subscriptions
> - Stick to one GP 'comic'
> - Skim the contents list (for future reference) of the journals
> - Limit yourself to one key article each week
> - Aim not to let a new journal into the house/consulting room without processing the previous week's first
> - Consider using the on-line versions (e.g. *BMJ*)

Particularly time-consuming are the Medical Attendant's Reports (MARs) for insurance and life assurance companies, which require a full review of the patient's medical records. As a GP registrar you should only do a few of these for practice. The same applies to private medical examinations for insurance or other purposes.

You will, however, have to do other letters and forms on behalf of patients you see in surgery although you will not be able to sign passport application forms as you must have known the person for at least 2 years.

Charging for extras

Many services, including completion of non-statutory forms, are not considered part of a GP's Terms of Service so the practice may charge a fee.* The practice will have a list of fees available at reception. Ask your trainer to go through the services that generate a fee to get an idea of the rates for the commonly used services so you can advise patients before you agree to undertake the task. This will save you and reception staff a lot of aggravation. In cases of patient hardship use your discretion to waive the fee.

* See Non-NHS income, p. 20.

Do not take money from patients yourself; direct them to reception who will issue a receipt, or pass the paperwork to whoever is responsible for invoicing and chasing up outstanding bills. Non-NHS fees generate a significant amount of practice income but do not worry if you fail to charge for something, particularly in your early days.

Dealing with requests for forms and letters

> - **Always obtain the patient's consent before releasing any medical information**
> - **Do not agree to sign or complete forms or letters you do not fully understand.**

Do not be pressurized into filling in forms or writing 'to whom it may concern' letters mid-surgery. Instead, ask the patient to leave the matter with you and complete it after surgery so you can give it proper attention. Give them a realistic timescale for its collection. If they want it sending then ask for a stamped addressed envelope. Advise them of any charge.

There may be an alternative to writing a 'to whom it may concern' letter. Housing departments often have specific forms to aid re-housing on medical grounds and will write to you for the information. They may ignore unsolicited reports.

If it is not clear what information is required ask the patient to have the third party write to you stipulating exactly what information they require.

Ensure all completed forms go through the practice administrator so that fees are collected. A copy should be kept in the notes.

Specific letter and certificate requests

It may be reasonable to refuse some requests. This will come with experience and confidence.

'Attendance at the surgery'

Practices may have a proforma ('This patient attended today') or you may need to write a letter. Some doctors refuse to issue such 'certificates' and request that the patient asks their employer or college to write to them directly. The GP will then confirm attendance in writing. This offer is, unsurprisingly, rarely taken up. Such requests are unreasonably using GPs to police the workforce and student population on behalf of employers and educational institutions.

Absence from school/college and sickness over exams

GPs are often asked to write certificates to cover a multitude of medical and non-medical situations to schools and colleges to explain short absences. Generally speaking the school should accept a parent's or student's word and not require a doctor's certificate.

Letters for illness during examination time are justified as they may be acknowledged by examiners and might affect grades.

'Fitness to ...' certificates

Patients may request certificates, and examinations, confirming their fitness for a range of leisure and work activities. This is to absolve an organization, such as a holiday tour operator, from responsibility should anything happen. However, the responsibility may then fall to you so beware.

Specific guidelines do exist on fitness to drive* and to fly as a passenger† or when pregnant (in which case advise the woman to contact the airline directly). For other activities you may feel insufficiently knowledgeable to confirm fitness. Unless the organization specifies the information it requires, or you know exactly what the activity involves and the level of fitness required, do not sign. Either refer the patient back to the organization or issue a general, non-committal letter such as: 'This patient is currently fit and well to my knowledge' or 'This patient suffers from X and is being treated with Y'.

* See Driving, p. 247.

† See Sources and further reading.

In some cases a full medical examination and completion of a certificate will be required and the patient will need to book an appointment specifically for this.

Holiday cancellation

The patient must have consulted a doctor at the time of the illness before you can confirm, for insurance purposes, an illness that necessitated holiday cancellation.

SOURCES AND FURTHER READING

1. The Cabinet Office. *Making a difference: reducing GP paperwork.* Report, March 2001.
2. Advising patients about air travel. *Drug and Therapeutics Bulletin* **34**(4): 30–32, 1996.
3. The Aviation Health Institute. *Contraindications to Air Travel: Guide for GPs*, www.aviation-health.org

16

Extras in the working day

INTRODUCTION

Aside from your basic clinical work there are many other elements to fit into the working day which can add stress if they are not antici- pated. To handle these extras you need to develop your time- management skills and your ability to delegate, and learn to say no from time to time. This is important to maintain good medical practice, avoid errors and protect your sanity.*

* See Looking after yourself, p. 78.

As with many other aspects of work your share of these will be much less than the partners, so use this time to establish good habits.

DAY-TIME DUTY DOCTOR

Between 7 a.m. and 7 p.m. weekdays each practice should have a duty doctor to deal with urgent calls and visits. You will be part of the duty doctor rota after an agreed period when you feel suitably confident and, of course, you should be supervised.

The duty doctor will be generally be responsible for:

- urgent visit requests
- urgent phone calls, prescription requests and abnormal results phoned through
- calls when the surgery doors are closed at times not covered by out-of-hours services (usually 7–9 a.m. and 6–7 p.m.). Encourage patients requesting visits at these times to come in to the surgery when they can be seen before or after surgery
- covering the surgery when it is closed in the day-time, for example lunch-time and afternoons.

Practices differ in how they divide up same-day urgent appointments. They may be passed to the duty doctor, or shared between all doctors working that day. Some practices reduce the amount of routine work arranged for the duty doctor to allow for the on-call work. The unpre- dictable nature of the work and longer working day can be pretty chaotic and stressful. Ensure you are well supported, delegate if possible and make time for meal and refreshment breaks. Leave your non-urgent paperwork until another day.

HIDDEN CONSULTATIONS

Patients increasingly communicate by letter, phone, fax and e-mail. Do not underestimate the work involved in these 'hidden consulta- tions' as they may include requests for prescriptions, referrals, forms for completion or other action. If it is clear that you cannot deal with the problem without seeing the patient, for example for a referral for a condition no doctor has seen or discussed previously, then ask a member of staff to call the patient and make them an appointment.

MANAGING INTERRUPTIONS

Interruptions are one of the more irksome parts of general practice, whether during a surgery (when patients deserve your undivided attention), paperwork session or coffee break. Although you are not at the end of a bleep, it can be harder to escape than in your hospital days.

If you feel you are having too many interruptions then discuss this with your trainer. Staff may be using you as a 'soft touch' as the new person in the practice, and you may need to firm up your boundaries.* * See Developing your boundaries, p. 77.

Interruptions from reception staff

Reception staff should not interrupt your surgery unless an emergency arises or they are having extreme difficulties with a patient. Medical emergencies and calls for truly urgent home visits are relatively rare. Social emergencies are not, for example needing a replacement Med 3 certificate, and although you should not always react immediately to these requests you will need to help out your battle-weary reception staff from time to time.

You may or may not be happy to be interrupted for calls from your nearest and dearest, so let reception know. Make clear the times when you absolutely cannot be disturbed, such as when you anticipate a difficult consultation, or simply need to blitz your paperwork.

Interruptions from professional colleagues

Do oblige your professional colleagues, particularly nursing staff, who need a second opinion or a prescription mid-surgery. You will need favours from them in return.

It is reasonable to take phone calls from other health-care professionals mid-surgery, especially if you have been waiting for them to phone you back. You should ask your current patient ' if they wouldn't mind waiting outside' to avoid breaking the confidentiality of the patient under discussion. Warn patients to expect an interruption if you are waiting for a call.

THE TELEPHONE AND MESSAGES

> **Document all phone consultations in the medical record with date and time.**

Make sure you know how to use the internal phone system.

Your practice should have a protocol for dealing with phone calls and messages left at reception from patients wishing to speak to a GP. There should be a set time before or after each surgery or even a phone surgery for this purpose. Receptionists should offer to help first, for example to chase appointments, arrange transport or contact expected district nurses, before asking the patient to call back or taking a message. Requests for prescriptions should not be taken over the phone.

The practice should have a watertight system for dealing with all messages from patients. Failure of such communication can lead to errors and complaints. There will usually be a message book, notes or e-mail directed to the relevant GP. Deal with your messages and return calls after each surgery, documenting all clinical contacts in the medical record with date and time. Ask patients to make an appointment if they launch into a lengthy phone consultation for a new problem.

Dealing with out-of-hours phone consultations is covered in Chapter 18: Out-of-hours work.

If there is no answer

Document failed attempts to return calls. Leave a neutral answer-phone message if possible: 'This is Dr ... from the ... surgery returning your call at 12.30 p.m. on Tuesday 4th January. Please call again if you still need to speak with a doctor'. Try again later if you consider the problem might be serious from the tone of the message left for you.

If you have serious concerns and are persistently unable to get through, discuss this with one of the partners. You may consider a visit to ensure the patient is alright. Very occasionally you will need to contact the police if you are unable to gain access.*

* See Home visits, if there is no answer, p. 172.

Phone calls from concerned relatives

These can be difficult to manage, particularly the 'please do not tell them I called' and 'I want to know what's wrong with my father ...' varieties. You must always protect your patient's confidentiality so explain that you cannot discuss your patient's care, even with family members, without their consent.† If necessary you should actively seek the patient's consent (by phoning them) and document this. If they do not want information to be disclosed you will have to pass this on to the

† See Maintaining confidentiality, p. 228.

enquirer. Alternatively suggest the caller make an appointment to see you together with the patient.

Difficulty accessing the practice by phone

Patients may complain to you that they cannot get through to you or the practice. Suggest they notify the practice manager as systems can be reviewed and changed. Dedicated appointments lines or specific times for accessing results may help. An answering service may be used midday to deal with emergencies. Whilst this allows practice staff to catch up with the morning's work it is not popular with patients.

MEETINGS

Although essential for management, service and educational aspects of working life (*Box 16.1*), meetings are often held at antisocial hours

---

Box 16.1   GP meetings

Practice administration
- Weekly practice meeting: day-to-day running of the practice
- Partner meetings: overview of practice and inter-partner issues
- Finance meetings: review practice accounts with accountant
- Away days: occasional meetings, for troubleshooting, team building or forward planning

Clinical
- Multidisciplinary PHCT to discuss shared patients
- Case conferences
- Mental health review

Educational
- In-house meetings: hot topic review, audit, outside speaker to discuss services
- Journal club
- Postgraduate centre meetings
- Self-directed learning groups including MRCGP study groups and non-principal or young practitioners' groups

Political/local planning
- PCG/PCT
- LMC

---

in order to fit into the overcrowded GP week. Ideally meetings should be well-planned, well-facilitated, kept to time and result in clear action plans to maximize productivity. Refreshments always help.

Attend weekly practice meetings, however irrelevant they may seem. They should provide good insight into practice management and partner relations and you will be expected to contribute. You may not be invited to finance or partners' meetings.

Try to attend both a child protection case conference and a multidisciplinary mental health team meeting of a patient you know during the year. Unfortunately these are often held at inconvenient times for GPs, such as mid-morning.

17
Home visits

INTRODUCTION

Home visits continue to form an important part of UK general practice both for routine and emergency consultations. GPs are variably enthusiastic about visiting. Consultations with patients in their own home can yield valuable information. You are more likely to make an appropriate OT or social services referral following a visit than a short surgery consultation. Although it is a privilege to be welcomed into people's homes, visits can be time-consuming, navigation and parking often frustrating and the home may not provide the ideal setting for a full clinical assessment.

PRACTICAL PREPARATIONS*

* See also, Your medical bag, p. 64.

Get to know your bleep for on-call days. Check you know how it switches on and off, the answering service number to call and where to find spare batteries. A mobile phone is essential.

You are required to have a car or other suitable transport for visiting. Parking regulations for doctors vary so check with your practice manager for local arrangements. Avoid identifying your vehicle as a doctor's to reduce break-ins. If you cannot get a replacement vehicle when yours is off the road then negotiate with your colleagues to undertake visits that can be done on foot.

SAFETY PRECAUTIONS (*Box 17.1*)

Personal safety is of increasing concern although cooperatives have considerably improved the safety of out-of-hours work.

Box 17.1   Visiting: safety precautions

- Always inform someone of the destination and expected duration of any visit you do unaccompanied
- Carry limited quantities of drugs and prescriptions
- Lock your car and your bag if left in the car
- Consider carrying a rape alarm
- Ask a family member to come out and meet you on unfamiliar housing estates
- Ask the police to meet you at the address if violence is a possibility

---

VISITS DURING THE WORKING DAY

Visit requests should be documented in the practice visit book. Most GPs visit at lunchtime so patients should make their requests in the morning by a stipulated time. Requests at other times will be passed on to the duty doctor and done before or after surgery. It is rare for a GP to need to leave mid-surgery for an emergency visit.

Visits 'in hours' are needed for the housebound elderly and chronically ill as well as those too unwell to come in (TCI) to the surgery. The non-housebound should be persuaded to attend the surgery if at all possible.

Regular visits may be scheduled to nursing or residential homes managed by the practice. Requests for visits may also come from Primary Health Care Team staff, particularly district nurses, when they feel a medical review is necessary for a patient they have been treating. Joint visits can be arranged with nurses or specialists such as psychiatrists, psychogeriatricians and the palliative care team.

Visits are usually distributed evenly among the visiting GPs for that day, although some practices stick to personal lists for visits and emergency consultations.* As a GP registrar you may cover absent partners' patients. Make sure you are not given more than your fair share. You may be allocated responsibility for a nursing home, which can be good experience. There will be days when you need to limit the number of visits you can undertake due to other commitments such as meetings and exams. Let your trainer know when this is the case.

* See Personal lists, p. 22.

AN APPROACH TO VISITING

Visit with your trainer for the first few weeks before visiting alone. As with all consultations, you should be supervised at all times by a named GP available by phone. Cooperatives are very specific about this requirement, which also applies to all 'in hours' visits you do.

Always inform reception and a GP colleague if you need to leave for a visit mid-surgery or will be delayed back for your surgery. They can appease, and perhaps see, some of your waiting patients.

Before you go

Phone the patient first to find out the exact problem and whether you need any specific equipment such as a nebulizer. Confirm the address and ask for directions. With experience you may be able to negotiate an alternative to a visit such as:

- attendance at the surgery in an urgent appointment
- telephone advice
- a prescription
- referral to a more appropriate health professional, such as a district nurse for a dressing problem.

If possible, speak to the patient's usual GP, or the district nurse or health visitor if they know the patient.

Ensure you have the medical records or a comprehensive computer summary together with an updated medication list. Let reception know where you are going and that you are effectively unavailable unless you are on call.

Most visits are to the elderly and so safety is rarely an issue, but if you anticipate violence from the tone of the request, arrange to meet the police there by phoning ahead to your local police station.

While you are there

Once you have found the place and introduced yourself, deal with the consultation much as you would in surgery. Be vigilant in keeping pets, and children's fingers, out of your bag. Ask to have the television turned off, toddlers tamed and distracting music turned down so you can concentrate on the consultation. Ensure you have good light and the patient in the best setting for a full examination, which may mean moving to another room. Remember to wash your hands after the examination, or use wet wipes in your car.

If you are unsure how to manage the patient then consider calling your trainer for advice from the patient's house or return to the surgery and call the patient back with a management plan.

Write up notes on site and leave prescriptions, investigation and referral paperwork with the patient. Make sure you take the medical notes away with you.

If there is no answer

Check you have the correct address, shout through the letterbox, or look through a window and phone from your mobile before assuming the worst (only to find they've gone to the hairdresser). Phone and discuss the situation with your trainer.

If there is no response and you have a high index of concern (based either on previous history or the reason for the visit request) consider calling your local A&E and the ambulance service to check if they are currently dealing with the patient. Only then consider calling the police to help you with access. Breaking the door down is rarely necessary. If you are less concerned then consider leaving a note, and phone the patient later.

On your return

Complete the computer and prescribing records. Write out FP10s to replace any drugs or dressings dispensed from your bag. Arrange any investigations and referrals, including to Primary Health Care Team members. Document future planned visits in the visits book and follow up any patients you are concerned about by phone at an agreed time.

SPECIAL CASES

Terminally ill patients

Looking after a patient through a terminal illness is a distressing but rewarding aspect of general practice, so try to get involved in the care of such a patient during your year. Patients can usually visit the surgery early on, but become housebound as their illness progresses. A weekly, or fortnightly, visit from the same doctor can be very reassuring to patients and their family. Always leave a good half an hour for such visits, have a cup of tea, and do not feel a need to 'do' anything beyond simple reassurance and acting as liaison between hospital, nursing and palliative care staff. A visit to bereaved relatives after a death is usually greatly appreciated.

Elderly housebound patients

Aside from dealing with the presenting complaint, use the visit for a general review including medication check, removal of obsolete medicines (with the patient's permission), giving a flu jab and health promotion advice. Check the patient has adequate support, identify any safety issues, such as loose carpets or need for bath rails, and make referrals for social services or occupational therapy input with the patient's agreement.

The acutely mentally ill patient

Even when a crisis is brewing and a mental health section possible, you may still be able to persuade a patient to come into the surgery, perhaps accompanied by their CPN. You will feel more secure at the surgery and have help more readily to hand.

If a section seems likely then accompany your trainer on the first occasion at least. Sectioning patients is covered in depth in Chapter 24: Clinical Issues with Legal Stipulations, The Mental Health Act and the Acutely Mentally Ill Patient, p. 250.

18
Out-of-hours work

INTRODUCTION

GP principals have a contractual obligation to provide 24-hour care to their patients. They can do their own out-of-hours work, delegate it to another GP, use a commercial deputizing service or share it with colleagues in a GP cooperative.

An annual payment is made to principals for providing this out-of-hours care and an item of service fee for each face-to-face patient contact between 10 p.m. and 8 a.m., even if their patient is seen by another GP. These payments can offset the costs of a cooperative or deputizing service.

There is an on-going debate as to whether the contractual obligation to provide out-of-hours care should rest with the patient's registered GP. There are also government initiatives to ensure all out-of-hours work reaches a minimum standard.

* See NHS Direct, p. 41.

The role of NHS Direct* is expanding as part of plans for an integrated national out-of-hours service incorporating GP services, walk-in centres, pharmacies, A&E, ambulance services and community nursing teams.

PROVISION OF OUT-OF-HOURS CARE

Out-of-hours typically covers 7 p.m. to 7 a.m. weekdays and around the clock on weekends and bank holidays. The duty doctor will cover the practice for emergencies between these times.†

† See Daytime duty doctor, p. 164.

There are several ways for practices to provide out-of-hours cover (*Box 18.1*). Some practices will use a combination of methods to achieve a balance between undertaking a reasonable workload without incurring excessive costs. There may be variations between partners in the same practice and some GPs delegate all their out-of-hours work. GPs may mix and match how they use services: they may speak to patients themselves then ask the cooperative or deputizing service to undertake any consultation or visit they decide is necessary.

Box 18.1   Providing out-of-hours care

- Own on-call
- Shared rota between practices
- GP cooperative
- Deputizing service
- Transferring responsibility to another doctor

Own on-call

An answering service (often through a cooperative or deputizing service) will take patient calls and bleep the on-call GP. The GP then phones the patient back and, depending on the patient's history, will give telephone advice or arrange:

- a prescription
- a surgery attendance or
- a home visit.

This procedure also applies to dealing with patient calls between surgery opening times and true out-of-hours (usually 7–9 a.m. and 6–7 p.m.).

GP cooperatives

These non-profit-making organizations are owned and staffed by local GP principals from several practices. The out-of-hours period is covered by 'base' and 'car' doctors, dividing the workload on a shift system and working from a primary care centre (PCC). This may be in a surgery, outpatient facility or A&E department. A car and driver, medical equipment and drugs are often provided and there is usually back-up from administrative staff. GP non-principals may also be employed, particularly to cover less popular shifts.

To access a doctor out-of-hours, patients phone their own surgery, and are either redirected to the cooperative or given the cooperative number on an answer machine message. Calls are triaged by a GP or nurse who will offer advice, consultation at the primary care centre or a visit. Details of the consultation are usually faxed through to the patient's practice for the next working day.

Cooperatives are funded by the member practices. These practices pay an annual fee for running costs and then work an agreed number of shifts depending on practice size. Alternatively they pay a fee for each patient contact and are paid for any shifts they undertake which allow practices to plan their workload to cover their bills. Some members may opt to pay for the service without undertaking any sessions themselves.

Deputizing services

These profit-making organizations offer an out-of-hours service, typically visits, but increasingly phone and surgery consultations, which are charged to the practice. They are staffed by employed or sessional GPs but not necessarily local principals. They also feed back to the practice usually with a note via the patient.

OUT-OF-HOURS AND THE GP REGISTRAR

> **You must always be adequately supervised when doing any out-of-hours work.**

Whilst cooperatives can be quite sociable, being on-call from home can be quite isolating and disruptive to your domestic or social life. Some people (and their co-habitees) deal better than others with being disturbed at home.

Your out-of-hours experience should give you confidence to:

- distinguish and manage the true medical emergencies from the many less urgent problems, including the social ones
- access other services including hospital specialists, ambulances, mental health, district nursing, pharmacy and social services out of working hours
- offer alternatives to home visits where you feel they are not necessary
- educate patients on the appropriate use of out-of-hours care.

It may be salutary to do the occasional overnight shift to see the different types of problems that arise and the responsibility that falls to you in the absence of other services.

If your practice uses a deputizing service then agree on a reasonable time to hand over to them in the evening when you are on-call for the practice, such as 11 p.m.

Your contractual involvement in and payment for out-of-hours work as a GP registrar is covered in Chapter 6: The GP Registrar Contract and Finances, Out-of-hours Work, p. 56.

GP registrar involvement in cooperatives

Each cooperative will have its own stipulations on how they involve GP registrars. The National Association of GP Cooperatives has produced guidelines intended to protect the GP registrar and reassure other GP principals that their patients are receiving a good standard of care.

You should not do any cooperative work alone for the first 3 months of your registrar year. Accompany your trainer until then. When you do go solo, which will usually be as the visiting car doctor, there must always be a named principal from your training practice available for advice or to come in if necessary. Ideally they should be working with you from the primary care centre.

Cooperatives may not allow GP registrars to do unsupervised telephone advice, although there should be opportunities to learn to consult by phone using a three-way or speakerphone facility with your trainer. You will also see patients who are invited in to the primary care centre.

CONSULTING OUT-OF-HOURS

---

1. Always take a thorough history of the presenting problem and ask specifically about:

- **concurrent medical conditions**
- **past medical history**
- **current medication**
- **allergies.**

2. Document all consultations with time and date.

The vast majority of patients use out-of-hours services appropriately for urgent medical problems that cannot wait until their surgery is next open. Most calls will be from parents with young children, the elderly and carers. There are many reasons for people to call, including having responsibility for someone else, a previous delayed diagnosis, fear about a specific illness (such as meningitis) or failure of self-treatment. Understanding patients' fears may help you reassure the caller and perhaps reduce your own exasperation at what you may otherwise consider a waste of time.

Requests for assessments may also come from district nurses, midwives and ambulance personnel.

Decision-making in emergency consultations

Use this useful algorithm (*Box 18.2*) in GP emergency contacts, in or out-of-hours.*

* See also Emergency referrals, p. 128.

An approach to out-of-hours phone consultations

Most out-of-hours consultations start with a phone call. Introduce yourself, clarify who it is you are speaking to and if it is not the patient then ask to speak to them as well if possible.

Use a general opener such as 'What can I do for you?' (even if you have some clinical details) and allow the patient to talk for a minute or two before you ask direct questions. Take into account how well, breathless or anxious they sound and make decisions accordingly (*Box 18.3*). If you cannot make a reasonable assessment over the phone then a face-to-face contact (as a visit or an invitation to the primary care centre) is essential. Those with poor English, learning difficulties,

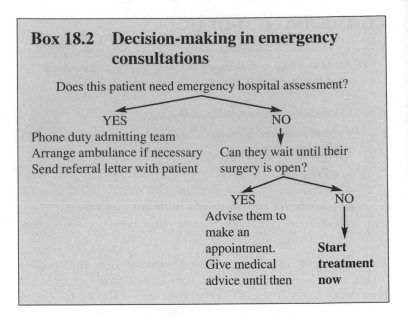

Box 18.2   Decision-making in emergency consultations

Does this patient need emergency hospital assessment?

YES
Phone duty admitting team
Arrange ambulance if necessary
Send referral letter with patient

NO
Can they wait until their
surgery is open?

YES
Advise them to
make an
appointment.
Give medical
advice until then

NO
**Start
treatment
now**

high anxiety or under the influence of drugs or alcohol can be particularly difficult to assess by phone.

If a patient calls back after initial advice then have a low threshold for a face-to-face contact. Let patients know if there will be a long wait for visits and request they call back should they deteriorate in the meantime. They may decide that they can make their way to you at the primary care centre.

Negotiating visits

Experienced GPs will try to discourage home visits when they are not clearly indicated. Patients will usually be seen quicker if they attend the primary care centre and it is a more efficient use of GP time. As a GP registrar you should not be solely responsible for declining visit requests when you work for a cooperative. Negotiating this takes practice. Observe how other GPs do this – it is a useful skill to learn: 'I think we should see you. Would you like to come in to …? You will generally not have to wait long. It is not like casualty! Let me give you the address and directions.'

If a patient insists on a visit that you deem unnecessary and a confrontation seems likely, then agree to the visit and save yourself stress. You should make it clear on the feedback to the patient's GP that the patient insisted. Children with fevers can go out, despite what parents believe. However the 'lack of transport' plea can be difficult to get round unless you work in a cooperative that arranges patient transport.

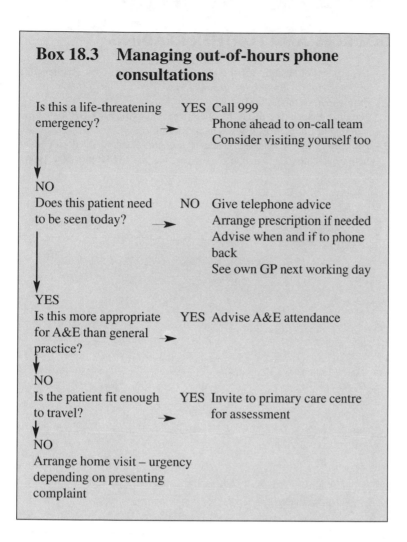

Box 18.3   Managing out-of-hours phone consultations

Is this a life-threatening emergency? ——→ YES Call 999
Phone ahead to on-call team
Consider visiting yourself too

NO
Does this patient need to be seen today? ——→ NO Give telephone advice
Arrange prescription if needed
Advise when and if to phone back
See own GP next working day

YES
Is this more appropriate for A&E than general practice? ——→ YES Advise A&E attendance

NO
Is the patient fit enough to travel? ——→ YES Invite to primary care centre for assessment

NO
Arrange home visit – urgency depending on presenting complaint

Using drugs out-of-hours

Avoid giving injections for chronic or recurrent self-limiting conditions such as migraine or IBS as this may encourage expectations of a repeat in the future. Buccal and rectal alternatives are usually available. Do not hesitate to use injections for severe chest pain, renal colic, intractable vomiting with dehydration and so on, pending transfer to hospital.

Chemists are usually open within 24–48 hours of an out-of-hours contact, so only give out starter doses of drugs.* Prescriptions can be phoned through to a local chemist,† but ensure that you have 'safety-netted' particularly well if you decide to do this.

* See also Ordering drug supplies, p. 69.

† See Prescribing over the phone, p. 105.

SOURCES AND FURTHER READING

1. Department of Health. *Raising Standards for Patients. New Partnerships in Out of Hours Care. An Independent Review of GP Out of Hours Service in England*, October 2000.
2. National Association of GP Cooperatives. *Guidelines for GP Registrars Working in Cooperatives*, www.nagpc.org.uk.
3. Hopton J., Hogg R., McKee I. Patients' accounts of calling the doctor out of hours: qualitative study in one general practice. *BMJ* **3131:** 991–994, 1996.

19
Educational aspects of the year

INTRODUCTION

The basic 12 months as a registrar will pass quickly and you are unlikely to fit in all that you would like. You may catch up with some of the elements you couldn't squeeze in, including the MRCGP exam, after qualification. Learning and training continues throughout your career so do not expect to master everything now.

Make the most of your study leave allowance and claim as much reimbursement as available.*

* See Claiming course fee reimbursement, p. 61.

Review and revise your plans regularly as the year pans out and keep in mind the bottom-line aims for the year when you feel distracted by other pressures:

- confidence to conduct a surgery safely and efficiently
- successful completion of summative assessment
- acquisition of your JCPTGP certificate.

The two big educational hurdles are summative assessment and the MRCGP exam. Although touched on in this chapter, we cover the requirements for these in detail together with some tips on how to approach them in the following chapters. We have devoted an entire chapter to the dreaded video.

Give yourself regular protected time, at home or work, for preparing tutorials, MCQ practice, and reading the journals.

SUMMATIVE ASSESSMENT AND THE MRCGP EXAM

Summative assessment is a test of minimum competence and successful completion of all four components is a requirement of your training. The MRCGP exam is considered a test of excellence and is not compulsory.

Although in your first few months as a registrar you will be busy orientating yourself clinically, start thinking about summative assessment and the MRCGP exam. An early start in preparing for these 'tests' should give you a feeling of control.

Plan your educational timetable with both these tests in mind. Ideally set your personal deadlines ahead of the official submission dates so you are always ahead of the game. You will actually absorb a lot of the knowledge you need from your day-to-day work, general chat in the surgery, and your VTS course. Start reading some of the more basic texts,† the journals and GP press early on.

† See Recommended reading, p. 279.

Both summative assessment and the MRCGP exam undergo constant development so always refer to the latest guidelines.‡

‡ See Chapters 5 and 20–22.

AIDS TO LEARNING

Adult learning

General practice training places a lot of emphasis on 'adult learning', that is self-directed, self-assessed and adapted to your personal needs with the help of a supportive tutor (your trainer), and other adult learners (your VTS group).

Although postgraduate education is often in lecture form, partly because this is relatively inexpensive, it is not always the most effective way to learn. The GP registrar year offers other means including personal tutorials, the VTS release course and small group study. Develop effective and time-efficient learning techniques now and you will find them invaluable for your future continuing medical education and re-validation.

Deanery educational pack

At the start of your year you should receive an educational pack (*Box 19.1*), together with a summative assessment pack, from your deanery office outlining local training requirements. Use the tools and topic lists to plan your tutorials and guide your preparation for summative assessment and the MRCGP exam. Ensure you have details of the local office website for training and education updates.

Box 19.1   GP registrar educational pack

- Educational contract
- Advice on learning methods
- Guidance on VTS release course and local educational opportunities
- Essential topics to cover and guidance on planning tutorials
- Weekly, monthly and annual planners for clinical and educational activities
- Logbook to record tutorial topics and educational events undertaken
- Self-assessment confidence rating scales and trainer appraisal forms
- Useful addresses and websites

Making the most of your trainer

Your trainer has many roles – as your tutor, colleague, mentor, role-model, counsellor, referee as well as employer. As a result the registrar –trainer relationship can be quite intense and probably unlike any other in your medical training.

Do not expect your trainer to be all-knowing; like the rest of us they have their strengths and weaknesses. Learn how best to use them and when best to ask for help.* Store queries up for the weekly tutorial where possible. Plan your tutorials together and review the topics list as you progress through the year. Remember that you must be supervised whenever you are working so reinforce the point if you feel 'neglected'.

* See Asking for help, p. 76.

Most registrars get on very well with their trainers and remain in contact when the year is over, although problems do occasionally arise. Try to discuss any problems directly with your trainer, perhaps after discussion with your VTS colleagues and course organizer. If you feel this is not possible or fails to produce results then approach your deanery. The regional BMA office may be able to help BMA members, especially for contractual and employment difficulties.

† Box 1.4, p. 10.

An outline of the general requirements for trainers and their practices is given in Chapter 1.†

Educational contract

This optional contract can supplement your employment contract and should be drawn up with your trainer. It should define the aims and objectives of your year, specify time for tutorials and study leave and provide a framework for planning your induction period, tutorials and assessments.

MAKING THE MOST OF THE EDUCATIONAL OPPORTUNITIES

As well as the more specific educational events there are continuous opportunities for learning in every aspect of your work (*Box 19.2*). Protected time and a structure for reflecting on what you have learnt will maximize the gains.

Box 19.2 Educational opportunities in the year

Surgery-based
- Surgeries
- Weekly tutorials with trainer or other partner
- Sitting in with and accompanying trainer or other partners and PHCT members
- Trainer sitting in with you
- Joint surgeries
- Practice meetings
- Complaints

Out of the surgery
- Visits
- Out-of-hours work
- VTS release course
- VTS residential courses
- Specialist outpatients
- Courses
- Local practice visits (negotiate with other registrars)
- Practice swap with contrasting training practice
- GP registrars' annual conference
- Postgraduate centre academic meetings
- Medical journals, GP press, circulars

Weekly tutorials

Devise a flexible programme of relevant topics with your trainer and keep a record in your logbook. Use the chapters in this book to provide a framework for your early tutorials and then be guided by your educational pack and clinical problems encountered in your work. It is important to ensure variety, so include:

- clinical topics
- management of difficult patients
- reviewing your videos
- discussion of ethical, legal, political and service issues.

Get your trainer to fill in the Structured Trainer's Report* as you go. * see p. 200.

Ideally both you and your trainer should spend time preparing for each tutorial to maximize the benefits. Your trainer should arrange for another partner to teach you if they are away.

VTS release course ('play school')

This is usually held during term-time at your local postgraduate centre and attendance is compulsory. Hospital GPs in training also attend. The course organizer devises the overall programme, ideally with your input (*Box 19.3*).

The format usually consists of a GP-relevant topic (with or without a speaker) and may include a discussion of problem cases brought to the group. Alternatively you may arrange a group visit to a local GP-relevant institution, for example a prison.

Be pro-active as a group and arrange the timetable and speakers. Pick subjects that interest or worry you. Prime outside speakers beforehand with questions and cases to focus them on your primary

---

Box 19.3 Suggested topics for VTS release course

Practical sessions
- CPR training and certification session (compulsory for the MCGP exam)
- Consultation skills (reviewing videos, rôle-play)
- Self-defence

Clinical topics
- Specialty update
- Substance abuse
- Eating disorders
- Complementary medicine
- Unfamiliar clinical topics

'Soft'/generic skills
- Communication skills
- People management
- Time management
- Financial and business management
- Stress management and preventing burnout
- Finding your practice and planning your future

Visits
- Local hospice
- RCGP
- Local prison
- Local practices

---

care needs. Limited funding may be available to reimburse speakers and the postgraduate centre should be able to set up equipment such as slides, overhead projector and video.

VTS residential

Most VTSs organize residential days or weekends away from the practice. These are usually held in pleasant surroundings (hotels) and focus on a particular GP theme. You should be able to obtain reimbursement for this as part of your study leave allowance. They are usually more fun than the prospect suggests, and a good excuse to escape the surgery, explore broader aspects of practice and bond with your fellow registrars.

Specialist hospital outpatients

Contact local consultants in the specialties you are interested in or ask your trainer to help organize some sessions for you at your local outpatients. Prepare a list of GP-relevant questions and cases you have seen in practice before you go.

Most consultants have great respect for their GP colleagues and are usually very obliging, but you may find yourself treated like a medical student.

Practice swap

These can provide a useful opportunity to get a taste of another type of practice. Ideally swap for a week with a registrar you know in another part of the country or working in a very different area or practice. Otherwise write to the Director in your chosen area for a list of training practices. Doing locums following your training provides similar experience.

GP registrars' annual conference

This conference is held by the GP Registrars Subcommittee of the GPC* and may be organized by a different region or VTS group each * See p. 41. year. It focuses on a political or practical GP theme relevant to registrars and involves talks, workshops and evening entertainment together with the usual drug company freebies and BMJ bookshop stand. Usually fun and painlessly educational, it is also approved for reimbursement.

Other opportunities

You can get involved in politics, for example representing GP registrars on the Registrars' Subcommittee of the GPC. Practice visits to inspect training practices usually include a GP registrar and can be an interesting afternoon out. Additional leave should be granted for these activities.

USEFUL SKILLS AND QUALIFICATIONS

Some skills and qualifications (*Box 19.4*) will broaden your scope for generating income for your future practice, entitle you to join 'health authority lists' and so make you more employable. All are useful (not compulsory) and GPs may actively decide against acquiring a certain skill, preferring to focus on other aspects of general practice instead. Approved regional courses are available for many of the practical skills. Select areas where you lack confidence as well as those that interest you. Aim for a good breadth of experience.

Box 19.4   Skills and qualifications for the GP registrar

- MRCGP
- Cardio-pulmonary resuscitation (compulsory for MRCGP exam)
- Child health surveillance (compulsory for MRCGP exam)
- Family planning (DFFP)
- IUCD insertion
- Minor surgery
- Diploma exams (e.g. Child Health, Obstetrics and Gynaecology and Geriatric Medicine)

MRCGP Exam Prerequisites

Cardio-pulmonary resuscitation and Child health surveillance certificates

Official proformas are issued with the exam regulations and are valid for 3 years from the date of signing. Further details are in Chapter 21: The MRCGP Exam.

Family planning and IUCD insertions

For the Diploma of the Faculty of Family Planning (DFFP) you need to attend a short course and then arrange at least eight practical sessions with a 'Faculty Instructing Doctor'. Look out for the theoretical courses locally in the medical press then contact your local family planning clinics or community gynaecology department for the practical sessions. Some clinics may charge you for sessions, including for coil training.

An annual fee is payable to the faculty for the DFFP for which you receive the regular *Journal of Family Planning and Reproductive Health Care*. Re-certification is required every 5 years. Full details and the official paperwork are available from the Faculty of Family Planning.*

For the Letter of Competence in Intrauterine Techniques (LoCIUT) you must have the DFFP and then accrue a minimum of 10 supervised IUCD insertions of at least two types of device. Some of these you may achieve in the practical sessions for the DFFP. You also need to be competent at assessing patients' suitability for IUCDs and dealing with coil problems. Again re-certification is required every 5 years but no annual fee is payable.

* See Useful addresses and websites, p. 273.

Eligibility for health authority lists

Health authorities hold lists of GPs (principals and non-principals) who have evidence of specific training in:

- obstetrics
- child health promotion
- minor surgery (including joint injections).

Such GPs can then claim additional payments (item of service fees) for services they provide. GP principals on the list can still claim fees even when the service is carried out by another GP not on the list, which includes you as a GP registrar.

Inclusion onto the lists is by application to the health authority, each of which have their own criteria. In general, proof of additional supervised clinical experience and/or attendance at an approved course is required. You cannot apply to be on a list yourself until you have finished your training, but it is worth getting the experience and funding for the relevant courses during your registrar year. Ask your practice manager to find details of your local health authority requirements, particularly if you are intending to work in the area on completion of your training.

Note that there are differing requirements for the Child health surveillance certificate for the MRCGP exam and for inclusion onto the health authority list for child health promotion.

THE DIPLOMA EXAMS

These optional exams (*Box 19.5*) 'recognize an interest' in a specialty and are useful to consolidate the experience acquired in your SHO jobs from a GP perspective. They are best done towards the end of or after each specialty post. They may be difficult to fit into the overcrowded registrar year so do not attempt to sit more than one in the year.

A minimum of 6 months' experience in the specialty is mandatory. They generally involve a written paper, which may only be MCQs, and a practical section that is either a clinical exam or an Objective Structured Clinical Examination (OSCE). They are held twice a year and several attempts are permitted.

All incur an exam entry fee (not reimbursable) and some an annual fee once you have got your diploma. It is worth attending a course before sitting the exam, for which fees may be reimbursable depending on local budgets.

Contact the individual Royal Colleges for details and application forms.*

* See Sources and further reading (below) and Useful addresses and websites.

Box 19.5   Diploma examinations

- Diploma of the Royal College of Obstetricians and Gynaecologists (DRCOG)
- Diploma in Child Health (DCH)
- Diploma in Geriatric Medicine (DGM)
- Diploma in Medical Rehabilitation (DMR)
- Diploma in Tropical Medicine and Hygiene (DTMH)

SOURCES AND FURTHER READING

1. Hall M., Dwyer D., Lewis T. *The GP Training Handbook*, 3rd edn. Blackwell Science, 1999.
2. London Deanery. *Assessment Toolkit* and *Study Guide for GP Registrars*. London Department of Postgraduate General Practice Education and Training, April 2001.
3. DFFP and LoCIUT regulations. Faculty of Family Planning and Reproductive Health Care of the Royal College of Obstetricians and Gynaecologists, www.ffprhc.org.uk
4. DRCOG Exam Regulations. Royal College of Obstetricians and Gynaecologists, www.rcog.org.uk
5. DCH Exam Regulations. Royal College of Paediatrics and Child Health, www.rcpch.ac.uk
6. DGM, DTMH, DMR Exam Regulations. Royal College of Physicians, www.rcplondon.ac.uk

20
Summative assessment

INTRODUCTION

This test of minimal competence was made compulsory for all GP registrars in 1998. Successful completion of all four components (see below) is a prerequisite to application for your JCPTGP certificate and thus your qualification as a GP in the UK.

Intended as a comprehensive assessment, it tests knowledge together with problem-solving, clinical, communication and written skills. Summative assessment aims to ensure basic clinical competence in all new GPs and to reassure the public that GPs are safe to practise. It should also identify doctors who would benefit from further training (or even another career).

The components do involve a lot of work (despite assurances given in the official documentation) and you may feel as though they detract from the clinical experience of the year. However it should not take over your life. You should have protected time for the written work component and support should be forthcoming from your trainer and VTS colleagues.

Components can be re-sat or re-submitted if necessary following input from your GP educators (trainer, course organizer, Director and/or summative assessment coordinator). Only about 4% of registrars do ultimately fail and further training can be arranged. Despite the low failure rate, the whole process can be rather anxiety-provoking.

ADMINISTRATION

Each deanery has a summative assessment office that will issue your summative assessment pack including a video pack, Structured Trainer's Report and practical guidance on completing and submitting the components. This office also administers the basic components and arranges the signing of your VTR/1 form when you have passed. Your national training number* should be entered on all submissions and correspondence.

Familiarize yourself with the latest national guidelines,† which should be included in your local office guidance.

Your Director will need to sign your VTR/1 certificate confirming you have passed all four components before you can apply for your JCPTGP certificate.

Your practice should provide all the equipment you need to undertake it and it should not cost you anything unless you undertake the MRCGP exam module options.

DEADLINES

You will need to structure your educational year around the exam dates and submission deadlines (*Box 20.1*), which you should have on your year planner.‡

* See Organization of training, p. 4.

† See Sources and further reading.

‡ See also The educational year, p. 50.

Box 20.1 Summative assessment year planner

Check also MRCGP exam submission dates

Month

1   Familiarize yourself with the requirements. Fill in the trainer's report as you progress

2 and 3 Start considering written work topic
Start videos for practice and improving consultation skills

4   Sit MCQ from now

5

6

7   Submit video or sit simulated surgery from now

8

9   Submit written work and video by end of month

10

11   Submit trainer's report by the end of the month

12   Get VTR/1 form completed by the trainer and Director
Apply for JCPTGP certificate

THE COMPONENTS

The four basic components are set by the Committee of General Practice Education Directors (COGPED). As the assessment has evolved more options are available, overlapping with the MRCGP exam in some cases (*Box 20.2*).

You also need to inform your local office of your chosen method for each component. As these cannot be changed you will need to decide early on whether or not to apply for the MRCGP exam.

You will need the permission of your Director to ensure funding for any non-COGPED components and you will have to pay for any MRCGP exam modules you opt for.

MCQ paper

The COGPED MCQ is a 3-hour paper, with 300 true–false MCQs and matched extended questions encompassing all modern general practice. It is held four times a year in each region and can be sat from month 4 of your GP registrar year onwards.

Alternatively you can sit the MRCGP MCQ paper, held twice a year. Your Director will need written evidence from the RCGP of your success in this to complete your VTR/1 form.

Box 20.2   Summative assessment
            components 2001

Component   **Method**
MCQ   • COGPED MCQ *or*
                           • MRCGP MCQ paper

Assessment of consulting   • COGPED video *or*
skills   • MRCGP video (MRCGP/SA
                             Single Route Video) *or*
                           • Simulated Patient Surgery

Written submission of   • COGPED audit *or*
practical work   • Project marked under the
                             National Project Marking
                             Schedule

Structured Trainer's Report

* See Chapter 21.

To prepare yourself use the topic list in your deanery educational pack and the MRCGP exam 'syllabus'.* Read up on and document (on index cards) unfamiliar clinical topics as you encounter them in surgery, read the major journals and practise MRCGP MCQs.

You can retake the COGPED MCQ, but after two failures you will need discussions with your GP educators. The current pass rate is about 94%.

Assessment of consulting skills

You can either submit a video or undertake the Simulated Patient Surgery. Ideally, both assessments should be submitted/undertaken in the final 6 months of training.

Video

You may choose to produce a video solely for summative assessment, or submit your MRCGP tape (MRCGP/SA Single Route Video). Full details of both are covered in Chapter 22: The Video. You should be sent a video pack including blank tape, guidelines, consent forms, summary sheets and a logbook for you to appraise each consultation.

Make sure you have advice from your trainer on the best consultations to submit from your many video-taped surgeries. You may submit your video between the end of months 6 and 9 as a GP registrar.

If your COGPED video submission fails you will be asked to resubmit another tape after a specific period of training. If this still fails you will need to discuss with your GP educators how to proceed.

Simulated Patient Surgery

These are held in real surgeries in South Trent and Yorkshire deaneries, usually in spring and autumn. Each surgery lasts about 2½ hours and involves eight consultations (of up to 10 minutes) with actors playing patients. You are allowed 5 minutes between consultations to complete a post-encounter form and the 'patient' also completes a satisfaction form and clinical checklist.

You must pass six consultations or you will need to undertake a further surgery. If you fail this you will be referred to an expert panel.

You will need to bring your usual diagnostic equipment and *BNF*. Familiarization sessions are organized twice a year and local workshops may be available. You must have permission from your Director to ensure funding is available should you choose this option.

Written submission of practical work

This can either be the COGPED audit or a piece of work that fulfils the National Project Marking Schedule (NPMS) criteria (see below). The work must relate to general practice and can be undertaken at any time throughout the 3 years of vocational training.

Although something of a chore, it can be quite rewarding to produce a piece of written work longer than a clerking or case presentation after leaving medical school, and publication might be possible.

Choosing a topic can be an initial stumbling block. Unless you have a burning interest in something, ask your practice for ideas as they will need audits for clinical governance. Failing that, brainstorm with your VTS colleagues and read the GP press for hot topics. Whatever you choose *keep it simple*. Ideally it should only take 10–12 hours work in total (*Box 20.3*).

Your practice should provide all you need to carry out the work and full guidance on how to present it should be available in your summative assessment pack.

Your written work must be submitted by the end of month 9 of the registrar year; that gives you enough time to re-submit it with amendments if necessary. If you fail you may need to submit an additional piece of work before the end of your training period or an extension of training may be needed.

COGPED audit

* See Clinical governance, p. 232.

Audit is a core component of clinical governance* and the ability to complete one is considered a skill of minimal competence. Your audit should involve a 3000-word report on a completed audit cycle written up under specific headings (*Box 20.4*) and three anonymous copies submitted.

National Project Marking Schedule

Under the NPMS other, more creative, self-directed work can be submitted (*Box 20.5*).

The project is intended to show that you can plan and sustain an activity and construct a logical argument written in clear English. Your planning and write-up should reflect the marking schedule so:

- State clearly the aim of your project or the particular problem or question you are investigating
- Reference relevant literature fully and include at least six references
- Describe your methods clearly so the reader could repeat the study. Write up the method before you collect any data
- Present your findings (qualitative or quantitative) clearly. Decide how you will present the results before you collect data and get external feedback on the clarity of your presentation
- Discuss your findings and include evaluations of how well your study addresses the question that you proposed

- Draw conclusions which should include practical suggestions for improvement.

Box 20.4   The COGPED audit criteria write-up

1. **What is the title of your audit?**
   Why did you choose it?
2. **Which criteria have you chosen?**
   Why did you choose them?
3. **What standards have you set?**
   Why did you choose these?
4. **What preparation and planning did you undertake?**
   First data collection   Date …
5. **How does this compare with your standards?**
6. **What changes are you implementing?**
   Second data collection   Date …
   Compare with data collection (1) and standards
7. **What conclusions have you drawn from this completed audit cycle?**

Reproduced with permission from the National Office for Summative Assessment.

The report should be between 1500 and 3000 words and four anonymous copies submitted.

**Box 20.5   National Project Marking
Schedule options for written work**

Options for submission

- Questionnaire study
- Notes review
- Literature review
- Clinical case study
- Research study
- Proposal for new service in the practice
- Audit
- Discussion paper

Box 20.6 The Structured Trainer's Report

Specific clinical skills
- Mental state examination
- Use of:
  - auriscope
  - ophthalmoscope
  - sphygmomanometer
  - stethoscope
  - peak flow meter.
- Vaginal examination
- Use of speculum
- Cervical smear
- Rectal examination
- Venous access
- Intramuscular and subcutaneous injections

Patient care
- Making a diagnosis:
  - communication skills
  - recognition of common physical, psychological and social problems
  - eliciting patients' beliefs, ideas, concerns and expectations
  - dealing with patient life events and crises
  - proficient examination of each system and organ.

Patient management
- Appropriate management of problems
- Management of emergency situations
- Care and support for patients and families
- Broad knowledge of all aspects of drugs

Organizational skills
- Clinical judgement:
  - appropriate examination
  - appropriate response to requests for urgent attendance.
- Organization:
  - awareness of personal limitations, appropriate referral and delegation
  - time management
  - understanding of contractual obligations of a GP.
- Professional values:
  - possession and application of ethical principles
  - maintenance of personal physical and mental health
  - accepting appropriate responsibility for patients, colleagues and others.
- Personal and professional growth:
  - identification of personal strengths and weaknesses.

CONTACTS

National Office for Summative Assessment	Ms Margareth Attwood Business Manager King Alfred's College Winchester Hants SO22 4NR Tel. 01962 827389
Simulated Patient Surgery: **Yorkshire Deanery** (for registrars in the northern half of the UK)	Mrs Carol Dobson Education Centre Strayside Wing Harrogate District Hospital Lancaster Park Road Harrogate HG2 7SZ Tel. 01432 554448
Simulated Patient Surgery: **South Trent Deanery** (for registrars in the southern half of the UK)	SPS Administrator General Practice Postgraduate Education Department University of Leicester Leicester General Hospital Gwendolen Road Leicester LE5 4PW Tel. 0116 258 8118
National Project Marking Schedule	The Administrator National Project Marking Schedule Department for NHS Postgraduate Medical and Dental Education (Yorkshire) Willow Terrace Road University of Leeds Leeds LS2 9JT Tel. 0113 233 1550

The Structured Trainer's Report (Box 20.6)

This report gives your trainer guidance on the minimum standards they should expect from you. The report is divided into six sections:

- patient care
- communication skills
- personal and professional growth
- organizational skills
- professional skills
- specific clinical skills.

Your trainer should assess you on these by:

- observation
- discussion and
- specific methods.

Go through this carefully with your trainer in your induction period. Your trainer should then fill it in on a regular basis throughout the year and may need a little prompting from time to time.

Aim to complete the clinical skills in the first part of the year, the patient care element as you prepare your video and your personal skills in the last 6 months when you should be evolving into an independent GP.

Professionals other than the trainer (e.g. members of the PHCT) can assess some skill areas. Some of the practical skills tested should really have been assessed at the end of house jobs rather than at this stage of your career.

Submission is due by the end of month 11. You will have several opportunities to demonstrate the skills (and learn from mistakes), but if your trainer has grave doubts about your ability to reach the required standard in all elements they will need to discuss it with you and inform your course organizer and Director.

SOURCES AND FURTHER READING

1. Committee of General Practice Education Directors. *Summative Assessment for General Practice Training.* August 2001 (also known as the 'Protocol'). Available at www.doctoronline.nhs.uk or in paper copy from the National Office for Summative Assessment, m.attwood@wkac.ac.uk
2. London Deanery Summative Assessment Guidance Pack, May 2001.
3. JCPTGP. *A Guide to Certification*, 2001.

21
The MRCGP exam

INTRODUCTION

This is an interesting, eclectic exam and encourages you to develop your own ideas on all aspects of general practice, health care and politics. Preparation for the examination allows you to consolidate your GP learning and get to grips with some of those elusive topics never quite mastered at finals and beyond. The exam should help you develop your critical faculties, structure your clinical thinking and begin to make sense of research papers in the major journals. You will have done much of the necessary work already for your summative assessment. Having MRCGP after your name should also improve your job prospects.

* See Royal College of General Practitioners, p. 42.

Taking the MRCGP exam is the main route to becoming a Member of the Royal College of General Practitioners,* the benefits of which may even be tested in a viva question. As a GP registrar you are eligible for associate college membership, which allows you the benefits of college membership including the monthly *British Journal of General Practice*, which is essential reading for the exam. New GP trainers must hold the MRCGP but established trainers are not obliged to acquire it.

This chapter serves as an adjunct to the:

† See Recommended Reading.

- exam regulations
- classic MRCGP texts†
- exam preparation texts† and
- specific courses.

It is not a guide on how to answer questions. Read it in conjunction with Chapter 19: Educational Aspects of the Year, Chapter 20: Summative Assessment and Chapter 22: The Video.

WHAT IS INVOLVED?

The exam is a four-part credit accumulation modular exam (*Box 21.1*) with two pre-exam requisites (*Box 21.2*), so you do not have to sit it all at one go. There is no strictly defined syllabus, but it tests what is thought to make a good general practitioner in the NHS today. The 'Domains of competence' determine the content of the modules (*Box 21.3*) and these are tested variously in each of the four modules.

Consult the latest examination regulations, which are available from the examinations department at the RCGP. They take a good while to digest. Information and news about the examination is posted periodically on the RCGP website.

Each module is held twice a year and can be taken alone or with other modules at the same sitting. Three attempts at each module are permitted, but all four modules must be passed within 3 years of application to pass overall, otherwise you have to start again. You need to make an application for the exam overall as well as for each individual module, and you pay for each module (£200 each in 2002).

The certificates of competence in both cardio-pulmonary resuscitation and child health surveillance must be submitted before you complete the examination.

Box 21.1   MRCGP examination modules

The written paper
- Modified essays on management of problems presented in UK general practice
- Critical reading: analysis and evaluation of published papers and extracts
- Knowledge of general practice literature
- Twelve or so equally marked short answer questions
- 3½ hours duration

The MCQ paper
- Up to 250 questions in a variety of formats
- 3 hour paper, machine-marked, no negative marking
- Covers:
  - medicine
  - administration and management
  - research, epidemiology and statistics.

Assessment of consulting skills
- Video recording of self-selected consultations

or

- simulated surgery consulting with a sequence of actors playing patients with defined roles
  Held in or near London, twice a year (only available to those with insuperable difficulties in making video recordings)

The oral exam (viva)
- Two consecutive 20 minute orals
- Each conducted by two examiners
- Emphasis on professional values
- Approximately five topics covered in each
- Covers:
  - care of patients
  - working with colleagues
  - social role of GP
  - doctor's personal responsibilities.
- Both orals similar in emphasis without significant reference to your own practice

---

Box 21.2   Pre-MRCGP certificates

Certificates provided in regulations book
Valid 3 years from date of signing
Must be submitted before you complete the exam

Proficiency in CPR
- Basic CPR
- Assessment by A&E or anaesthetic consultant, GP with special interest in CPR, Resuscitation Training Officer, etc.
- Holders of ALS certificate issued within last 3 years exempt

Child health surveillance
- Specific surveillance tasks include: developmental check/examination on 6–8 week old, 6–9 month old, and 3–4 year old
- Health promotion
- Immunization advice
- Assessment by GP principal on health authority child health surveillance list, community paediatric consultant, clinical medical officers working for a health authority, *not* health visitors
- Attendance at a theoretical child health promotion course alone is *not* sufficient

Box 21.3   Domains of Competence tested by the MRCGP examination

- Factual knowledge
- Evolving knowledge: uncertainty, 'hot topics', qualitative research
- The evidence base of practice: knowledge of literature, quantitative research
- Critical appraisal skills: interpretation of literature, principles of statistics
- Application of knowledge: justification, prioritizing, audit
- Problem-solving: general applications
- Problem-solving: case-specific, clinical management
- Personal care: matching principles to individual patients
- Written communication
- Verbal communication: the consultation process
- The practice context: 'team' issues, practice management, business skills
- Regulatory framework of practice
- The wider context: medico-political, legal and societal issues
- Ethnic and trans-cultural issues
- Values and attitudes: ethics, integrity, consistency, caritas
- Self-awareness: insight, reflective learning, 'the doctor as person'
- Commitment to maintaining standards: personal and professional growth, continuing medical education

WHEN TO SIT IT

The MCQ and video are worth getting out of the way during the registrar year together with the CPR and CHS certificates. Processing the current literature and mastering critical appraisal requires a lot of work and may be better deferred so it does not interfere with the clinical work of the year. Try to start your study group with your VTS colleagues during the registrar year.

Some choose to do the exam immediately after the GP registrar year and do locums rather than full-time work to ensure free time for study. You will usually have colleagues from your VTS doing it at the same time. Other GPs prefer to leave it until later, but run the risk of never finding the ideal time. Experienced GPs are usually more confident with the 'difficult patient', practice management and ethical aspects than GP registrars or the newly qualified.

There are two sittings a year, usually May and October, with the orals about 6 weeks after the written papers. Applications have to be in several months before the exam, around January for the summer sitting and July/August for the winter sitting.

WHO CAN TAKE IT

Independent practitioners of general practice or those undergoing vocational training are eligible. Even if you pass the entire exam during your GP registrar year you will not be granted full college membership until you have received your JCPTGP certificate.

HOW TO APPROACH IT

Although you will probably have absorbed enough basic knowledge throughout the year to pass the exam, applying this knowledge for the requirements of the individual modules and ensuring you are up to date with the current literature is what presents the challenge. This is where exam preparation books, courses and your study group are essential.

The following will help your preparations:

- Read both GP and non-GP texts. Anything with a remotely health and social care, ethical, organizational, educational or political flavour will be useful and will keep your mind ticking over. Include the daily non-medical press and novels
- Learn the skill of critical appraisal (how to read and analyse a paper) early on

- Go through the current literature and identify the 'hot topics'. Use the GP press as well as the standard journals
- Develop an approach to the written questions on clinical management and practice management and organization
- Practice viva questions.

Keep summaries of key facts, main reference papers and contentious issues together with your frameworks for answering the different types of question on filed index cards.

Organizing your study group

Aim for a group of between three and six members. If you are attempting the exam well after your training then contact the local VTS to find out who is doing the exam. They may well welcome a more experienced GP.

When to start depends on how you are intending to pace the modules but consider at least 3 months' preparation for covering the current literature.

Meet fortnightly initially, then weekly in the run up to the written papers and vivas. Make it convivial, but be focused. Spend a reasonable amount of time planning how you will run the meetings and prepare a list of likely topics to include clinical problems and broader general practice themes. Use the group to share out the hard graft preparation for the hot topics as well as practising the different types of written and viva questions.

Each group member should focus on an individual topic, research the information and then produce a handout summary for everyone. Cover:

- a revision of basic facts
- new developments
- application to clinical practice
- summaries of key papers
- future developments and
- contentious points.

Present and discuss the topics at the meetings. If you master critical appraisal early it will make interpretation of papers much less daunting.

Current literature and 'hot topics'

The hot topics are likely to come from the previous 18 months' main journals (*Box 21.4*), so focus your journal searches on these, but also

Box 21.4   Sources for Hot Topics

Hot Topics in General Practice – summarizes papers on key GP themes (Ese Stacey, BIOS Scientific Publishers)

Journals
- *British Medical Journal*
- *British Journal of General Practice*
- *Drug and Therapeutics Bulletin*
- *Evidence-Based Medicine*

Others
- National guidelines
- RCGP occasional papers
- RCGP information sheets
- Seminal papers on important topics

look out for notable articles in the *Lancet* and *New England Journal of Medicine*. Recently published research papers are often summarized and commented on in the GP press so it is worth reading these before you confront the original research paper. You will need to be aware of seminal past research papers that have influenced key developments in general practice.

Do not forget to cover major recurring topics (coronary heart disease, diabetes, NHS reorganization, etc.) and do not rule out covering topics just because they have featured in recent exam papers.

You should be able to mention references from reputable journals and books in your answers, but it is not essential to quote results and references precisely. It may be enough to give an indication that you have heard or read something about the latest developments on a subject.

Past papers and work books

Sample questions are included in the examination regulations. Past papers are also available from the RCGP (for a fee), but they do not contain answers. There are also published books of MCQs and critical reading, with guidance on how to approach the questions. Ensure you use an up-to-date text reflecting the current exam format.

MRCGP courses

Critical appraisal and the oral exams worry most candidates, so it is worth attending a course that demystifies these. Courses should give

* See p. 43.

guidance on how to answer the written questions and may question-spot. The Royal Society of Medicine,* RCGP and regional faculties run courses. Ask your course organizer and RCGP local faculty office; otherwise keep an eye out in the *BMJ* and *British Journal of General Practice*. Fees should be reimbursable.

The video

Preparation for this is covered in the next chapter.

ONCE YOU HAVE PASSED

Congratulations!

You can only use the letters MRCGP once you have your JCPTGP certificate and have paid the annual subscription fee. This is usually kept at a low rate for the first 5 years of membership, can be paid in instalments and is tax-deductible.

MEMBERSHIP BY ASSESSMENT OF PERFORMANCE

Introduced in April 1999, MAP provides an alternative means of achieving college membership. It is intended primarily for established GPs who do not have the time available for the intensive study involved in the examination. Those eligible must have at least 5 years' eligibility to work as a GP and be working at least three sessions a week in general practice in the year before application. MAP shares with the exam the requirements of assessment of consultation skills (by video or simulated surgery) and submission of CPR and child health surveillance certificates. However the other skills are tested by completion of a workbook and a day-long practice visit by two external assessors. It is actually more expensive than the exam and may take between 6 months and 3 years to complete. Bear this in mind if you vowed never to do another medical exam after summative assessment.

SOURCES AND FURTHER READING

1. RCGP. *Examination for Membership (MRCGP) Regulations*, 2002, www.rcgp.org.uk
   See also the Recommended Reading section.

22
The video

INTRODUCTION

With the introduction of summative assessment and the incorporation of video assessment into the MRCGP exam, videos of the consultation have become an inescapable part of formal GP training. There is little doubt about the educational value of reviewing video recordings to develop your consultation technique, but producing an edited tape of good consultations with pertinent commentary can be a time-consuming and anxiety-provoking task. Video-taping surgeries can certainly make them more stressful, at least initially, due to:

- the extra effort made to consult particularly well
- technical hitches and
- securing patient consent before and after the consultation.

So here we offer some practical tips to ease the process.

You will need your trainer's help together with the classic consultation texts and latest summative assessment and MRCGP exam regulations. The University of Birmingham Department of General Practice has also produced some video training packages to help with preparation for both summative assessment and the MRCGP. Check if there are any local courses available.

GETTING USED TO THE PROCESS

Seeing and hearing yourself on screen – particularly in professional mode – is pretty excruciating for most of us. The good news is that the more you do the easier it gets, so start to video a few consultations early in your year (about month 2). Do not wait until you can consult 'perfectly'. This will help you get used to the process and technicalities even if your are unconfident (and embarrassed) about your consulting skills. It can also be illuminating to compare early tapes with consultations later in the year. When you feel more confident start video-taping with the requirements of both summative assessment and the MRCGP exam in mind (see below).

Reviewing your taped consultations

Review your tapes regularly and soon after you make them (hours of accumulated surgeries to review is a pretty daunting task). View your consultations on your own to start with, then use tutorial time to discuss them with your trainer and make your selections for submission for summative assessment and the MRCGP exam. At some stage you may feel confident enough to expose yourself to your VTS group, which can provide invaluable feedback.

Pendleton and colleagues suggest a damage-limiting approach to reviewing consultations with others (*Box 22.1*).

Box 22.1   Guidelines for appraising consultations

Pendleton rules
- Briefly clarify matters of fact such as drug doses, follow-up or urgent consultation
- The doctor in the video makes the first appraisal, then other viewer/s
- Good points first – positive points commented on initially, such as manner, body language, open questioning
- Recommendations for change (not criticisms) should follow – with the consulting doctor commenting first, for example, missed possible hidden agenda

---

As you develop confidence analyse the consultations using the criteria for summative assessment and MRCGP (see below). This way you can see if you frequently miss any competences.

REQUIREMENTS FOR THE SUMMATIVE ASSESSMENT AND MRCGP EXAM VIDEOS

The requirements for video assessments undergo constant re-evaluation and amendment so always refer to the current regulations.*

A single tape† will suffice for both assessments provided the MRCGP-focused consultations are first on the tape. A pass in the MRCGP will be accepted as evidence for competence in consulting skills for summative assessment. If you are using the same tape for both, send your tape and paperwork to your summative assessment office (not RCGP) by the specified dates and they will forward it to the RCGP. If you fail the MRCGP module the tape will be returned and fast-tracked through the summative assessment process.

Consultations must demonstrate the skills being tested (*Box 22.2*) so do not use 'no challenge' consultations such as repeat pill requests or short follow-up consultations. Not all consultations have to show all the competences. The criteria for both tapes are fairly similar (*Box 22.3*).

* See Sources and further reading.

† The MRCGP SA Single Route Video.

Consent forms, a logbook with your appraisal of each consultation and a summary of the contents of your tape should be included with your video submission.

> ## Box 22.2 Competences to be demonstrated on video
>
> **Summative assessment**
> - **Listening**: identify reasons for attendance; arrange mutually acceptable management plans
> - **Action**: take appropriate steps to identify, investigate, manage and refer problems, and organize a suitable management plan
> - **Understanding**: logbook completion to show understanding of process and outcome of consultation, including any shortcomings
> - **Errors**: avoidance of major error (causing actual or potential harm to patient) or minor errors (causing inconvenience)
>
> **MRCGP Exam**
> - Discover the reason for the patient's attendance
> - Define the clinical problem(s)
> - Explain the problem(s) to the patient
> - Address the patient's problem(s)
> - Make effective use of the consultation
>
> Each of the above is broken down into 'performance criteria' or PC, demonstration of which results in a Pass or Merit point
> If sufficient criteria are not seen in the first five consultations next two will be viewed

PRACTICALITIES

Basic equipment

Your practice must provide all the video equipment (*Box 22.4*) you require for summative assessment.

Most training practices should now own cameras, otherwise borrow one from the VTS.

Box 22.3 Comparison of video requirements

Summative assessment

- See latest summative assessment guidelines

- Two hours of complete consultations, a minimum of eight consultations

- Maximum 15 minutes per consultation

- In English (Welsh if it is patient's preference but other consultations must be in English). Logbook must be in English

- Good sound and picture quality. Both doctor and patient's face visible

- No intimate examinations to be seen. Examination couch out of view (sound recording to continue)

- No clinical content specified

- Use standard summative assessment/MRCGP consent form

- Submit consent form and completed log entry with summary for each patient

- Submit log of contents of final tape with timing of each consultation

- Submit by end of month 9

- Pass or fail, but re-submission possible

MRCGP Exam

- See RCGP Video workbook and instructions for up-to-date requirements

- Seven complete consultations (first five will be assessed initially)

- Only first 15 minutes of consultation will be assessed

- In English

- As summative assessment

- As summative assessment

- Must include:
  - one consultation with child under 10
  - one with significant psychological or social dimension.

- As summative assessment

- As summative assessment

- As summative assessment

- Submit by, or on, date of written papers (twice a year)

- Pass with merit, pass or fail

Box 22.4   Video equipment

- Video camera, ideally with:
  - tripod or wall mounting facility
  - lens cap/shutter with on-going sound recording
  - remote control
  - built-in and remote microphone
  - day, date, timer counter with on-screen display
  - playback on the camera.
- Several blank tapes for the camera
- VHS tape supplied by your Summative Assessment Office, and blank 120 minute tapes for MRCGP exam and personal copies
- VCR player to edit/record from the camera
- Consent forms (photocopy 40 or so)
- Practice information leaflet if necessary
- Clipboard and pens at reception

A standard VHS tape is required for submission so you will need to copy from the smaller camcorder tapes (VHS-C) via a VCR. Do not record on long play. Make at least two other copies of your final tape.

Setting up the camera

Spend an early tutorial collecting video equipment and familiarize yourself with the basic workings of the camera. Get a demonstration (and read the instruction booklet). Have a dummy run with a member of the practice staff and make a test recording each time you set up your equipment (*Box 22.5*).

Box 22.5   Setting up the camera

- Ensure both you and the patient are in the frame
- Do not have the camera facing direct light/windows (close blinds and use artificial lighting)
- Check sound quality:
  - use an external microphone (ideally suspended rather than lying on desk)
  - keep windows closed/fans off.
- Ensure date/timer display are on
- Ensure you have enough film in the camera

Preparing the consulting room

Reduce clutter on your desk and ensure any visible shelves are not bare. Re-arrange the furniture, if necessary, so both you and the patient are visible. Make sure the examination couch is out of view but where this is not possible keep the camera running with the lens cap on when examining patients. If you have re-located to another consulting room for filming then familiarize yourself with its layout and get rid of other doctors' ephemera. Have a clock visible on your desk if your camera does not have a built-in timer.

PLANNING

Organizing video surgeries

Start by video-taping a couple of consultations each surgery, then plan to do a weekly video surgery once you are relatively confident in your consultation and camerawork skills. Vary your video day: Friday afternoon general practice can be very different from Wednesday mornings.

Let reception know which these surgeries are so they can block out slots or increase your appointment time. Good consulting and technical hitches take time and some patients may use consultation time discussing the video process itself. Involve reception staff fully and be sure they understand why you are making videos. This should help them to encourage, but not bully, patients to consent (see below). Patients should be informed about your intention to video both when they book an appointment and when they turn up. Receptionists should hand out the consent form, with pen, before the consultation but you may prefer to get the post-consultation consent yourself as the receptionist may miss the patient leaving. Ask reception staff to minimize interruptions.

Avoid taping the same patient more than twice, even though some patients seem to like it.

Aim to tape at least three to four times as many consultations as you will need to give you a good pool to select from. Many of your recordings may be unsuitable for technical, not clinical, reasons (see 'pitfalls' below).

Consent and maintaining confidentiality

Consultations may only be filmed with explicit informed consent that must be written consent signed both *before and after* the consultation on the standard consent forms provided (same one for both summative assessment and MRCGP). The form should be copied for the patient's medical record and reference should be made that the consultation was recorded. Anyone accompanying a patient who appears in the video should also give consent and forms should be available in languages other than English.

Most patients are happy to be filmed to help with teaching and training, but the opportunity to decline should always be offered. Confidentiality, the reason for the video and who will be viewing the tape should be emphasized. Patients should also be offered an opportunity to view the video. Some patients, such as non-English speakers, refugees and those with mental illness, may need extra explanation.

A named doctor, usually your trainer, should be responsible for the security and the confidentiality of the recordings and tapes should be stored with the same security as medical records (if not more). You should leave them in a locked cupboard or drawer. Be vigilant if you view your tapes at home. All recordings should be destroyed one year after the date of consent.

Taping the consultation

You may decide to tape the entire surgery, leaving the tape running throughout, but this can waste tape, especially if you are called out of the room frequently. It is also pretty tedious to review. You must, however, tape the entire consultation, which includes bringing the patient into your room. Ensure you have the correct patient's notes visible and their details up on the computer before they enter. You may find patients take a few moments to establish where the camera is. Be ready to turn off the camera at any point at the patient's request (it is useful to have a remote control). It is fine to film 'non-intimate' examinations, such as those with the patient in the chair, or standing, but not intimate ones so remember to take off the lens cap or open curtains afterwards.

Ideally the patient should sign the post-consultation consent form at reception. You can film your request for post-consultation consent, although it may feel like it interferes with the flow of a normal consultation.

Pitfalls

However well your surgeries seem to go there are often unpleasant surprises when you come to review your tapes. You can learn from our mistakes (*Box 22.6*).

Box 22.6   Video pitfalls

- Overbooking video clinics
- Forgetting to put on the timer
- Running out of tape mid-consultation
- Catching only part of the patient's or doctor's face
- Seeing too much of an intimate examination
- Lighting and noise 'pollution'
- Failure to get post-consultation consent
- Overlong good quality consultations

PREPARING YOUR FINAL TAPE FOR SUBMISSION

Do not underestimate how long this can take. You need to:

- review your taped surgeries
- select technically and clinically suitable consultations
- get an independent assessment of your selections (ideally your trainer)
- edit onto a single VHS tape with the MRCGP consultations first if appropriate
- make at least two other copies
- analyse the content of each consultation and complete the summary forms, keeping copies
- complete the log of the tape with accurate timing.

For the final tape you may wish to record a short introduction such as: 'My name is Dr ... and I am making this recording for summative assessment and the MRCGP exam.'

Go through the final checklists for summative assessment and MRCGP exam before submitting the tape. Ensure you have numbered the consent forms appropriately, included one for each consultation and filled in the summaries legibly. Deliver the final product (in a protective padded envelope) personally, or by Royal Mail Special Delivery or courier and then breathe a huge sigh of relief until the results come through!

SOURCES AND FURTHER READING

1. Committee of General Practice Education Directors. *Summative Assessment for General Practice Training,* August 2001 (also known as the 'Protocol'). Available at www.doctoronline.nhs.uk or in paper copy from the National Office for Summative Assessment, m.attwood@wkac.ac.uk
2. RCGP. *Video Assessment of Consulting Skills in 2002. Workbook and Instructions,* www.rcgp.org.uk
3. Pendleton D., Schofield T., Tate P., Havelock P. *The Consultation.* Oxford University Press, 1984.
4. Skelton J., Field S., Hammond P. *et al. Watching Me, Watching You. Consultation Skills and Summative Assessment in General Practice.* University of Birmingham Department of General Practice and West Midlands Postgraduate General Practice Education Unit. Radcliffe Medical Press.
5. Skelton J., Field S., Wiskin C. *et al. Those Things You Say ... Consultation Skills and the MRCGP Examination.* University of Birmingham Department of General Practice and West Midlands Postgraduate General Practice Education Unit. Radcliffe Medical Press, 1998.

Introduction to medico-legal aspects of general practice

> **Have a low threshold for contacting your medical protection organization for advice on any legal, ethical or professional practice matter.**

As a GP you will be more directly exposed to patient complaints and potential litigation than in your hospital posts where you are protected by the trust, NHS indemnity and your senior colleagues. This greater exposure is reflected in the steep rise in your medical protection organization subscriptions, fortunately most of which are refunded during the registrar year.*

* See Medical protection organization subscriptions, p. 59.

That complaints and legal action against doctors are generally on the increase is probably due to a combination of factors including:

- increased patient awareness
- greater availability of medial information and
- an increasingly 'consumerist' attitude to medical care.

Medical mishaps also make good press, which is often rather wearing to a demoralized profession. In light of recent disasters the medical profession itself, through the GMC and BMA, and the government are increasing surveillance and regulatory procedures for all doctors. Revalidation throughout one's career will soon be in place in an attempt to identify poorly performing doctors early and hopefully make rehabilitation a realistic option.

PREVENTING COMPLAINTS: KEEPING YOURSELF INFORMED

Even if you are extremely clinically astute and conscientious, problems can often arise from poor communication, medication errors or practice system failures. Worse still you can be tripped up simply because you are not aware of the legal stipulations surrounding practice, some of which we touch on here and by which you should abide. Some of these legal stipulations will be derived from statutes (acts of parliament stating clear requirements, which may not be solely medically relevant, such as the Data Protection Act 1998), others are derived from case law (principles derived from the interpretation of individual court cases applicable to all areas of clinical practice) or codes of conduct or statements of professional responsibility issued by the GMC.

The law is constantly evolving so you will need to keep yourself informed by:

* reading your GMC guidance booklet*
* availing yourself of advice booklets from your medical protection organization*
* keeping an eye out in the GP and medical press for relevant changes in the law
* buying a text on the legal aspects of medical practice.

You should practise defensible, not defensive, medicine (which is exhausting, inefficient and probably damaging to the doctor–patient relationship) so you should be aware of the pitfalls and how to avoid them.

* See Sources and further reading for Chapters 23 and 24.

23
Guidance for good professional practice

INTRODUCTION

Our aim in this chapter is to help you avoid making mistakes in your clinical care and reduce complaints against you and your practice.

Broadly speaking, there are issues for which you are individually responsible and those that are the responsibility of the practice. Although rather detailed we make no apologies for overstating the 'bottom lines'. You are probably already abiding by these principles and will only need to refer to this, and the next chapter, to confirm this in difficult situations. When potential problems do arise, always discuss them with your trainer and get in touch with your medical protection organization early.

Most of these principles and legal requirements apply to the law in England and Wales only, so check national variations.

We also look at how to cope should you receive a complaint against you.

DUTIES OF A DOCTOR

Familiarize yourself with the guidance from the GMC (*Box 23.1*), with which you must comply as an obligation of registration.

UNDERSTANDING CONSENT

A patient's consent, that is their agreement to undergo an examination, investigation or procedure, is required in any medical interaction (*Box 23.2*), although the nature of consent and the documentation required as evidence of the consent depends on the actual situation.

Failure to obtain appropriate consent can lead to a claim for and potentially recovery of damages (see below) either through a civil action for battery or a criminal action for common, aggravated or indecent assault. However, a few situations exist where consent is not required, such as treatment authorized under the Mental Health Act, some immigration and psychiatric examinations, and treatment ordered by a court.

For terminations of pregnancy or sterilization procedures consent is required from the patient only. It is good practice to seek to involve the patient's partner in the discussion but only with the patient's full agreement.

In difficult situations you will need to seek advice from your trainer, colleagues and possibly your medical protection organization.

Box 23.1 GMC Duties of a Doctor

Patients must be able to trust doctors with their lives and well-being. To justify that trust, we as a profession have a duty to maintain a good standard of practice and care and to show respect for human life. In particular as a doctor you must:

- Make the care of your patient your first concern
- Treat every patient politely and considerately
- Respect patients' dignity and privacy
- Listen to patients and respect their views
- Give patients information in a way they can understand
- Respect the right of patients to be fully involved in decisions about their care
- Keep your professional knowledge and skills up-to-date
- Recognize the limits of your professional competence
- Be honest and trustworthy
- Respect and protect confidential information
- Make sure that your personal beliefs do not prejudice your patient's care
- Act quickly to protect patients from risk if you have good reason to believe that you or a colleague may not be fit to practise
- Avoid abusing your position as a doctor
- Work with colleagues in the way that best serves patients' interests.

In all these matters never discriminate unfairly against your patients or colleagues and always be prepared to justify your actions to them.

Reproduced with permission from GMC, Duties of a Doctor, booklet series.*

* See Sources and further reading.

Nature and validity of consent

Three conditions must be satisfied to ensure consent is valid:

- the patient must have the capacity to give consent (see Competence below)
- they must have sufficient information to make an informed choice
- the consent must be given voluntarily.

Consent may be implied, such as by presentation at the surgery for a medical examination, or given expressly. You should be careful not to misinterpret a patient's apparent compliance as consent. The patient

> **Box 23.2   Clinical situations for which consent should be sought**
>
> - All clinical examinations
> - Intimate examinations (rectal and vaginal) and always offer a chaperone
> - Investigations including simple blood tests
> - Treatments including injections, minor surgery procedures (suturing, joint injections), radiographic procedures and major surgery
> - Passing on medical information to any third party*
> - Others sitting in on the consultation (students, trainees, other health professionals, patients' friends, relatives, translators, health advocates)
> - Photographing or video- or audio-taping patients
> - Entry into clinical trials
>
> *Third party includes a patient's relatives, spouse, employers, insurance company and publications.

should always be fully informed before they can give consent so you must explain any procedures and treatments you intend to carry out. Confirm with them that they have enough information to make a decision and document your discussion.

Oral consent should be sufficient for most procedures carried out in general practice, such as venesection, but for more complex procedures (typically minor surgery) you should obtain written consent. Although there are actually few situations where it is legally imperative to obtain written consent, for example for some fertility treatments, documented consent provides evidence that it has been obtained and may be useful should there be a future challenge. Many surgeries produce their own written consent form for minor surgery procedures, but this is, at best, only some evidence that consent has been obtained.

Competence (the capacity to make decisions)

Any competent adult can give or refuse consent, and every adult should be assumed to be competent unless proven otherwise.*

For an adult to be considered competent they must:

- be able to understand treatment information which should be presented clearly

* For which guidance is available from the BMA in conjunction with the Law Society – see Sources and further reading.

- believe it *and*
- retain it long enough to weigh it in the balance and make a decision.

Under-16s and 'Gillick competence'

A child can consent to medical treatment themselves if they are 'Gillick competent', that is they have sufficient understanding and intelligence to enable them to understand fully what is proposed including what is involved and its possible consequences. A competent child can also refuse treatment but this can be overridden by a parent or court if it is considered in the child's best interests (except in Scotland, where different rules apply). Such situations are difficult and you should seek legal advice.

Several individuals can also consent on behalf of a child:

- anyone with parental responsibility (automatically the mother and, in specific circumstances, also the father, other relatives or social services) and
- a court if necessary.

Where contraceptive advice and treatment are concerned, under-16s can be seen and treated without the consent of their parents if the treating doctor feels they are competent. You should encourage parental involvement but it is not obligatory, and you should reassure the young person that they will be seen in confidence.

Refusal of consent

A competent adult is entitled to refuse consent (to treatment, investigations, admission, etc.) and no one else can give consent on their behalf. A competent pregnant woman can refuse any treatment even if this course of action would be harmful to the foetus.

If a competent patient's choice seems irrational to you, or not what you would consider to be in their best interests, then you should review whether they have enough information to make that decision. If they still refuse then respect their wishes.

You have a duty to explain fully all the implications of rejecting the proposed intervention and offer the best available alternative to which they will agree.* Document the interaction fully.

* See also Patients refusing emergency referral, p. 129 and Patients refusing tests, p. 140.

Treating incompetent adults: 'best interests' principle

No one can give consent on behalf of an incompetent adult who cannot make their own decisions. However the patient can be treated in their 'best interests' without their consent. Any such treatment should be limited to that which saves life, ensures improvement or prevents deterioration in their physical or mental health. This decision should take into account any advance statements of refusal by the patient,* knowledge of their background and input from those who know them well.†

* See Advance directives, p. 238.

† See also The Mental Health Act and the acutely mentally ill patient, p. 250, on treating mentally ill patients who refuse treatment or are unable to make a decision.

Emergency situations where consent cannot be sought

In such situations the 'best interests' principle above should be followed, with treatment limited to that which is immediately necessary. You should tell the patient what has been done and why as soon as they are sufficiently recovered.

Where parents refuse consent for a child in an emergency situation but a doctor considers it in the child's best interest to go ahead, then the child can be treated. Again, seek legal advice in such situations.

Temporary incompetence

Patients may be treated in their best interests without their consent in situations of temporary incompetence such as those induced by needle phobia or severe pain.

Examinations for medico-legal purposes

Such examinations (for the police, or solicitor) still require a patient's consent unless there is a court order or authority under the Police and Criminal Evidence Act. Again, always seek advice from your medical protection organization.

MAINTAINING CONFIDENTIALITY

Confidentiality is central to ensuring trust between doctors and patients. The easiest ways to breach patient confidentiality are by casually discussing patients where you can be overheard and by leaving medical records (paper or electronic) where they can be seen, so always be on your guard. You should be aware of the principles of the Data Protection Act 1998.‡

‡ See Protecting patient information, p. 123.

You must always obtain consent from the patient or someone authorized to act on their behalf, before disclosing any medical information about them, unless you are referring them to another healthcare professional for treatment and the patient has agreed to the referral (*Box 23.3*).

Box 23.3 GMC principles of confidentiality for disclosing medical information

- Seek patients' consent to disclosure of any information wherever possible, whether or not you judge that patients can be identified from that disclosure
- Anonymise data where unidentifiable data will serve the purpose
- Keep disclosures to the minimum necessary

Patients should understand what will be disclosed, why and to whom and the consequences of disclosure.

Reproduced with permission from GMC, Guidance booklet: Confidentiality: protecting and providing information Paras 1 and 14

It is important to make it clear to spouse, relatives and friends that you cannot discuss a patient's medical case without the patient's express consent.* You should reassure your patients of this.

* See also Phone calls from concerned relatives, p. 166.

If you do decide to disclose any information without a patient's consent (see situations below), then you must be prepared to explain why and justify your decision. Always seek medico-legal advice if you are unsure.

Disclosing medical information

To employers and insurance companies

GPs are regularly asked for information and reports about their patients for such third parties which can only be released with the patient's signed consent. The third party will usually send the signed consent form to the GP together with the request for the report.†

† See Form-filling, letter-writing and other certificates, p. 158.

Patients are allowed to see such reports before they are sent out, under the Access to Medical Reports Act 1988 (*Box 23.4*). Most patients will not want to see the report and indicate this on the consent form provided. As with accessing medical records,‡ a GP can refuse the patient access to the report if they believe it would be likely to cause serious harm to the patient's physical or mental health.

‡ See Patient access to medical records, p. 118.

In other circumstances

If a patient refuses to give consent to release information but you believe the disclosure is in their best interests, then you may do so. Again, be prepared to justify your decision. Discuss such cases with your trainer and medical protection organization and document the matter fully.

Box 23.4   Access to Medical Reports Act 1988

- Concerns only reports written by doctors responsible for the patient's care for employment and insurance purposes
- Allows patient access to the report before it is sent to requesting party
- Patient's application to see report must be made within 21 days of report being written
- Copy of report must be provided to the patient if requested
- Patient may discuss the report and request an amendment (codicil) for incorrect or misleading statements provided that the GP agrees (patient could ultimately refuse release of report)
- Amendments must be declared on the form
- Copy of the report must be kept by the GP for 6 months from completion, whether the patient wishes to see it or not

Where a patient lacks the capacity to consent to disclosure of information (through immaturity, illness or mental incapacity) then try to persuade them to allow an appropriate person to be involved in the consultation. If this fails then act as above in their best interests. Inform the patient beforehand that you are going to release information without their consent.

In cases of neglect, and physical or sexual abuse, where the patient is unable to give or withhold consent, then information may be released to a statutory body or responsible person in order to prevent further harm to the patient.

In the interests of others

Disclosure of information without a patient's consent may be necessary if failure to do so puts other patients, or the public, at risk of death or serious harm, for example where patients continue to drive against medical advice.* Such disclosure should be done promptly to the appropriate person or authority.

* See Patients refusing to disclose to the DVLA, p. 249.

Where a doctor colleague (or patient of yours) is placing patients at risk as a result of their illness or another medical condition you are also obliged to take steps.

For the prevention or detection of a crime

Consent from the patient is still required for disclosure of medical information to police, solicitors and officers of the court unless a court order requests disclosure of such information or the public interest in disclosure outweighs the duty of professional confidence. Seek advice if you find yourself in this very unusual situation.

After a patient's death

There remains an obligation to keep information confidential after a patient's death, but this varies with circumstances. You may need the consent of the patient's executor, who should be fully informed as above. This is relevant where a life assurance company wishes to know the details of a patient's death before they agree to pay out. Again, seek advice.

REDUCING RISKS IN CLINICAL MANAGEMENT

Although much of this is covered in Section D, Day-to-Day Clinical Work of the GP Registrar, it is worth reiterating a few principles here:

- Keep full, legible and up-to-date notes. Document, document, document after any clinical patient encounter. Remember to date and sign entries, and add the time for difficult, emergency and out-of-hours encounters
- Keep patients and any health professionals involved in their care fully informed, unless the patient asks you not to
- Be meticulous when you prescribe*   * See Chapter 10: Prescribing.
- Adopt accepted practice: follow guidelines, especially evidence-based ones, where they exist
- Act within your limitations: look things up, ask for help or refer as necessary
- If you delegate then be sure that whoever you delegate to is up to the task.

On a lighter note, apparently American doctors who communicate well and laugh and joke with their patients are less likely to be at the receiving end of a malpractice lawsuit. Take heed.

RESPONSIBILITIES OF THE PRACTICE

Ensuring good systems are in place

Watertight systems should be in place for:

- reviewing repeat prescriptions
- reviewing and acting on results

- ensuring follow-up
- passing on messages
- making urgent referrals and
- flagging up allergies, for example.

Ideally these systems should be devised by the staff who are involved in them and reviewed regularly.

You should have comprehensive introductions to the practice systems in your induction period. You should also feel comfortable about letting your trainer know if you feel a practice system needs tightening up. This could be a good starting point for your audit.

Clinical governance

This was introduced in 1999 by the Department of Health in order to maintain high standards and safeguard quality within the NHS. PCG/PCTs are responsible for establishing clinical governance in primary care (*Box 23.5*).

Box 23.5 Components of clinical governance

Clinical and organizational audit	Reviews whether a process conforms to a predetermined standard
Risk management	Aims to reduce the likelihood of adverse events affecting staff and patients
Evidence-based practice	Good quality evidence to support clinical practice
Quality improvement	Monitoring and measuring performance against standards
Personal and organizational development	Individual development and training focusing on care to patients
Obtaining patients' and users' views	Develop partnership with the public
Measures for tackling under-performance	Essential for all practices to have systems for managing under-performance either internally or with external support

---

In practice clinical governance means practices must develop health and safety protocols, organize regular audits and review adverse events, amongst other things. With the support of local PCG/PCTs, local guideline initiatives and audit support groups, practices in a given area can work towards common goals and standards.

COMPLAINTS

Complaints are an inevitable part of practice and happen to everybody; both authors received complaints in their registrar year and are still here to tell the tale. Mistakes will always be made, even with the best will in the world, so be prepared to deal with the consequences. Clinical governance aims to reduce risk and provide a framework for managing mistakes when they occur, in a move towards a culture of openness.

If you have made a mistake

We all make mistakes, clinically or administratively, but fortunately most do not have significant impact on our patient care. If you know you have made a mistake then be honest, with yourself initially (often difficult), and then discuss the matter with your trainer. You may need to seek advice from your medical protection organization. You must be open and honest with the patient, apologize, and make amends if necessary, as soon as possible.* It can be quite a relief to share these errors with your VTS colleagues. You will find that you are not alone.

* See also Defusing a potentially violent situation, p. 90.

Practice complaints procedure

The NHS introduced a new format for handling complaints in 1996 (currently under review) and the system for general practice can be divided into three levels:

- level 1 – practice-based complaints procedure
- level 2 – independent review at health authority level
- level 3 – health service commissioner – ombudsman.

All practices are required to have a documented complaints procedure that you should read. When a patient makes a complaint they should be given a practice leaflet explaining this procedure and offered an appointment to discuss their complaint confidentially, usually with the practice manager or nominated partner. They should receive a response within 10 working days.

Few complaints go beyond the practice complaints procedure and it is rare for complaints to lead to claims of negligence (see below).

The health authority may refer cases directly to the GMC or even the police, if professional performance is seriously deficient or fraud suspected. Patients may decide not to use the NHS complaints procedure but consult a lawyer directly instead, or do so having used the standard complaints procedure. If a complaint is made against you and legal bells are sounding then contact your medical protection organization immediately.

Dealing with a complaint against you

If you receive a complaint, discuss it with your trainer or another partner as soon as possible. Consider contacting your medical protection organization depending on the nature of the complaint.

Review the medical records and write down anything further that you remember at this stage, for your own records. Do not be tempted to alter the records.* You may also need to write an official report.

* See Amending medical records, p. 117.

Follow the practice complaints procedure and be prepared to meet the patient, together with one of the partners and the practice manager. Listen to the patient, apologize if appropriate and provide reassurance that measures will be taken to avoid the mistake being repeated.

Even if the complaint is unfounded you should still allow the patient a chance to air their grievances and you may need to clear up any misunderstandings. Remember that patients may make complaints because they are angry or feel let down, so you may need to exercise some of your consultation skills in trying to help them express this.

Coping with a complaint

Complaints can be devastating for the individual doctor concerned. They often appear a long time after an event and can catch you completely off-guard. No one responds well to complaints and doctors may respond particularly badly, perhaps because of the potentially serious consequences of mistakes we make. The agony can also be prolonged by protracted investigations and procedures.

Expect to feel crestfallen, have your confidence shaken and have a few sleepless nights. You will probably find yourself being extra vigilant for a while afterwards. *It is vital to seek support, from medical colleagues and others, and to try to put the matter into perspective.* Remember all the times when things have gone well – keep a record of gifts and thank you letters to reflect on at times like this.

Learn what you can from a complaint: it does not necessarily mean you were in the wrong and need to change, but there is always something to learn. Essentially you will not please all of the people all of the time however hard you try.

If you feel you are receiving more than your fair share of complaints discuss this with your trainer. You may need to spend some extra time improving your clinical knowledge and developing your consultation skills.

CLINICAL NEGLIGENCE

Given that this is probably something most of us live in dread of being accused of and sued for, here are a few, hopefully reassuring, words. Negligence is a legal concept which implies that a reasonable standard of care was not achieved and that this is proven by a responsible body of professional opinion. It does not imply that the error was made on purpose or through active neglect.

In order for a negligence claim to be successful and damages paid all the following prerequisites must be fulfilled:

- the doctor owed a duty of care to the patient (you establish a duty of care whenever you enter into a therapeutic relationship with a patient)
- the doctor was in breach of that duty
- the patient suffered harm *and*
- that harm was caused by a breach of the duty of care (which can be hard to prove).

Damages (compensation) are payable to rectify the harm caused by the error. The amount is calculated to restore the claimant to the position they would have been in had the negligence not occurred, to compensate for loss of earnings, for care required and so on.

Your medical protection organization subscription should protect you against all the financial implications of such litigation. If negligence is clear, and the defending doctor agrees that the patient suffered harm as a result of a breach in the duty of care, then an out-of-court settlement may be made.

SOURCES AND FURTHER READING

1. Knight B. *Legal Aspects of Medical Practice*, 5th edn. Churchill Livingstone, 1992.
2. Marquand P. *Introduction to Medical Law*. Butterworth Heinemann, 2000.
3. Palmer K.T. *Notes for the MRCGP*, 3rd edn. Blackwell Science, 1998.
4. BMA and The Law Society. *Assessment of Mental Capacity: Guidance for Doctors and Lawyers*, 1995.
5. GMC. 'Duties of a Doctor' booklet series:

- *Good Medical Practice*, May 2001
- *Seeking patients' consent: the ethical considerations*, November 1998
- *Confidentiality: protecting and providing information*, September 2000
- *Serious communicable diseases*, October 1997
- *Management in Health Care: The Role of Doctors*, December 1999
- *Maintaining Good Medical Practice*, July 1998

6. Medical Protection Society. *Managing the Risks in General Practice.* MPS, 2001.
7. Panting G. *Consent to Treatment.* Medical Protection Society, 1999.
8. Panting G., Halliman E. *Dealing with Negligence Claims: a Member's Guide to Procedures in England and Wales.* Medical Protection Society, 1999.
9. NHS Executive. *Clinical Governance. Quality in the New NHS.* Department of Health, 1999.
10. Department of Health. *Acting on Complaints.* Department of Health, 1995.

24
Clinical issues with legal stipulations

INTRODUCTION

This chapter covers clinical issues with a specific medico-legal background that you may have touched on in your hospital practice already. We re-visit these issues here because, as a GP:

- you are more exposed to complaints and litigation
- patients will benefit from your advice on these issues
- they may crop up in the MRCGP exam.

In some cases we offer a clinical management framework, but this should not be taken as definitive guidance. Discuss these issues in your tutorials and follow up some of the recommended further reading. The order of the topics covered is purely alphabetical.

ADVANCE DIRECTIVES

Also known as advance statements and living wills, these written statements allow for a legally competent* and adequately informed individual to refuse specific treatment at a future time when they may no longer be competent.

* See Competence (the capacity to make decisions), p. 226.

These statements are legally binding so long as the individual made the decision voluntarily and there is no reason to believe that they would have changed their mind between making the statement and the relevant clinical situation arising. Patients cannot legally request a particular treatment, although they may authorize or refuse treatments.

When managing a patient who is not legally competent, doctors should make efforts to find out if an advance directive exists (drawn up when they were competent) and they should abide by any advance refusal if a specific clinical situation has occurred.† Problems can arise if the directive does not apply specifically to the patient's current condition or the instructions are vague, in which case treatment should probably be given in the patient's best interests.†

† Full GMC guidance in their booklet: *Seeking patients consent: the ethical considerations: para 22.*

‡ See Treating incompetent adults: 'best interests principle', p. 227.

GPs may be involved by helping patients draw up these documents or witnessing a patient's signature. Copies should be kept in the patient's medical record, which should be marked to this effect. Model advance directives are available from The Terrence Higgins Trust and the Voluntary Euthanasia Society.*

* See Sources and further reading.

CHILD PROTECTION

> *If you suspect child abuse then discuss it with your GP colleagues initially and report it to social services or a paediatrician. You could be considered negligent for failing to do so.*

Dealing with suspected child abuse is stressful for all involved so familiarity with the legal frameworks, key personnel (*Box 24.1*) and local protocols should help you develop a systematic approach to managing such cases. It is always a difficult issue as there are unpleasant implications for everyone involved, including the effects of a possible false accusation, but you will never have to deal with a case alone, even after your training. Spend a tutorial discussing the management of a real or fictitious case.

Abuse includes physical, emotional and sexual abuse as well as neglect and Munchausen by proxy. Consider it where there is a vague story, odd parental behaviour, failure to thrive or unusual injuries and discuss your concerns with your colleagues. Retain a low threshold of suspicion for referral. Abuse may take a while to come to light through suspicions of all those involved in child-care, including teachers. Aside from alerting the authorities and ensuring the child is safe, you do not always have to act in a hurry. Your area will have a Child Protection Team or Committee including social services, doctors, health visitors and the police, which is responsible for managing child abuse and which you will be able to contact via social services or the community paediatric team. They will be responsible for updating local protocols, a copy of which should be available in your practice.

Box 24.1   Key players in child protection

Children and families social workers
- Statutory duty to investigate cases of suspected abuse
- Your first point of contact
- Will check initially to see if a child is already known to them or on the Child Protection Register (see below)
- Main role is to protect the child and support the family
- May contact you for medical information on a child reported to them by the school or even the police

Health visitors
- Can keep an eye on families to follow up any low-grade suspicions
- Involved in case conferences
- Practice should have regular review meetings with them to discuss families of concern

Paediatrician
- Area lead paediatrician, usually a community paediatric consultant
- Responsible for dealing with suspected and confirmed abuse cases
- Often involved in detailed sensitive examinations, particularly where sexual abuse suspected
- Should be available to discuss individual suspected cases with GPs

The Children Act 1989

> **Treat the child's interests as paramount**

This Act stipulates that the welfare and wishes of the child are paramount, particularly where court decisions are involved, and that children are to be kept informed and involved in decisions about their future. The law emphasizes that the best way to protect their welfare is to support the care of the children within their family unless this is not in their best interests. Removing a child from the family should never be undertaken lightly.

Action in suspected abuse

If a child is medically at risk, due to serious injury, burns or neglect, then refer them to hospital immediately. Make your suspicions of abuse explicit to the on-call paediatricians who should then refer to social services. Document fully your suspicions and referral in the medical record.

In less acute cases follow the Child Protection Committee protocols. Contact the duty social worker in the first instance. You (or the social worker) may involve a paediatrician for a further skilled assessment. Keep detailed notes. Always put the child's immediate medical and emotional needs first. Arrange treatment for medical problems. Even if the child is not seriously injured a brief hospital admission may be required for assessment and observation or to remove them from a dangerous situation.

Keep the family fully informed throughout. Parents often feel very threatened at the prospect of social services being involved, so take time to explain that you are making the referral to support the child and the family. Stress that intervention to remove the child is not usually a priority. If parents refuse to allow you to involve social services, discuss the case with your trainer and medical protection organization before acting without their consent. Remember that the welfare of the child is your main concern.

Case conferences

Less urgent decisions about the child's future are often made by multi-disciplinary case conferences. GPs may be invited to attend these with members of the Child Protection Team and other involved professionals. They are often held during surgery time so it may be difficult to attend, in which case you may need to prepare a report. The outcomes of the conference may include:

- placement onto the Child Protection ('at risk') Register (see below)
- the need for a court order (see below)
- a Child Protection Plan for the future
- arrangements for review after an agreed period.

Criminal proceedings may be undertaken against the perpetrator if abuse is proven.

Child Protection Register

These registers are kept by social services and hold information about children suffering or likely to suffer significant harm. Details of the type of abuse suffered, a personalized Child Protection Plan and names of key workers involved are included. The register has no legal standing but signifies both the level of concern and need for monitoring. Decisions to place and remove a child's name from the register are made in case conferences and the GP and health visitors should be informed whenever a child is added to or removed from the register. Medical records should be updated accordingly.

Emergency Protection Order

This court order allows a child to be removed from their normal residence or stipulates the circumstances under which a child can be seen (such as by a parent). Application for the order is usually made by social services but doctors and the police may also apply. The order is effective immediately and without notice to the parent, lasts for 8 days, and can be extended for a further 7 days.

Police have separate powers to remove children to suitable accommodation when there is good reason to believe they may experience significant harm otherwise. Doctors may need police to invoke this power in order to admit a child to hospital where a child needs medical attention. The power lasts for 72 hours.

Other GP involvement in child protection

GPs have a vital role in supporting the child and family during and after investigations of abuse. Families may become divided both geographically and emotionally as a result of suspicions or revelations of abuse.

DEATHS

You are more likely to encounter unexpected deaths and possible suicides in the community than during your hospital experience and you are more likely to involve the coroner. You will also be involved in supporting the deceased's family in the immediate bereavement period and beyond.

Here we consider only the statutory requirements and practicalities following a death; palliative care and the bereavement process should be covered in depth in your tutorials.

Practical tips

- Accompany your trainer or other partner when they are dealing with a death so you can see through the process of confirmation of

death, certification and liaison with the next of kin, funeral directors and coroner
- Forewarn colleagues and the out-of-hours service of any imminent expected deaths of patients under your care
- When you are asked to confirm an unexpected death of someone you do not know, ask for clinical details of the deceased and who will be there when you arrive. The police, as the coroner's representatives, will often be present at the scene
- Debrief with your trainer and VTS group if you are involved with a difficult death

Confirmation of death

Be thorough with the usual examination (*Box 24.2*). Ask relatives if they would like to leave the room so you can do a full external inspection without feeling rushed or distressing them further. Look and feel for pacemakers in case a cremation certificate is required. Document full details in the patient's medical record together with the time of your examination and the time of death if known (ask the relatives).

Box 24.2   Confirmation of death

- No spontaneous respiration
- Pupils fixed and dilated
- No carotid pulse
- No heart or breath sounds over 1 minute

Death confirmed at ...
Time of death as reported to me ...

If you are working out-of-hours and the deceased is not a patient of yours or your practice, then inform the family they need to contact the deceased's GP, who may be able to issue the death certificate (see below) and with whom you will have liaised. Remember to phone or fax that GP, so they are aware of the situation before the family get in touch.

Removal of the deceased

How this is done depends on whether or not the coroner is involved (see below) after death is confirmed:

- If the coroner does not need to be involved, then the body can be removed by a funeral director, usually available on-call 24 hours. The next of kin then collects the death certificate from the patient's GP, takes it to the Registrar of Births, Deaths and Marriages, who then issues the Order for Disposal required by the funeral director before burial or cremation can proceed.

Some elderly patients and those with terminal illness may well have made prior funeral arrangements. Carry the contact details of a local funeral director in your on-call paperwork for the relatives of those that have not.

- If the coroner is involved then the body must not be moved until assessed by the coroner's officer who will arrange removal of the body (often to the local hospital mortuary). The coroner may then organize a post-mortem if necessary and issue the death certificate, after which the family can proceed with funeral arrangements.

Issuing the death certificate

A death certificate ('Medical Certificate of the Cause of Death') is usually completed by the patient's GP so long as certain prerequisites are fulfilled (*Box 24.3*), otherwise the coroner must be informed. If you are unsure whether you can issue the certificate then discuss it with the coroner's officer, who will usually be very obliging.

Box 24.3 Prerequisites to issuing a death certificate

- Cause of death must be known
- There is no need to report the death to the coroner
- The doctor completing the certificate has attended the patient in their last illness and seen them within 14 days of the death

The following do not matter:

- Which doctor confirmed the death as long as the details are known to the certifying doctor
- That the certifying doctor has not seen the body after death (although this may change in line with other European countries).

Reproduced from Knight, *Legal Aspects of Medical Practice*, 1992.

Your practice will have a book of death certificates with counter-foils. Complete these legibly and in full, avoiding vague causes of death such as 'old age'. Many causes of death are incorrect compared to post-mortem findings. You need only add your basic medical qualification to your signature, and put the surgery address under the 'your residence' section. Document the death certificate entry of causes of death in the patient's medical records. You may need these details to complete a cremation form later.

Try to complete the certificate as soon as possible after the death out of courtesy to the relatives. Some religions have stipulations about burying the deceased within 24 hours of death so you may find yourself under some pressure to complete the certificate mid-surgery. Deaths must be registered within 5 days in England and Wales and Northern Ireland or 8 days in Scotland unless the coroner is involved.

Informing the coroner

Suspicious deaths, deaths where the cause is unknown and others (*Box 24.4*) should be reported to the coroner. This is usually via the coroner's office during working hours or at your local police station out-of-hours. About a third of deaths are reported, but not all will require a post-mortem.

If you do inform the coroner then always tell the relatives and the reasons why. Forewarn them to expect a visit from the coroner's officer to avoid undue alarm at 'police involvement'. Out-of-hours cooperatives may have a policy of reporting all out-of-hours deaths to the coroner's officer who will then liaise with the patient's registered GP on the next working day.

Cremation certificates

Cremation is usually less expensive than burial. Only two of the eight forms for authorizing cremation are relevant to GPs.

Form B

Familiar from your hospital days, this is completed by the doctor who completed the death certificate. There is a statutory obligation to view the body after death so if you confirmed the death you can complete the form at the surgery. If not you will need to arrange with the funeral directors to view the body and complete the form there. This may involve a visit before surgery or at lunchtime. Take the patient's medical records with you for reference. Remember to feel for pacemakers. Some GPs undertake pacemaker removals for which they receive a fee.

Box 24.4 Deaths to be reported to the coroner

- Where cause of death is unknown
- Sudden death
- Deceased not attended by a doctor in their last illness
- Deceased not seen by the doctor completing the death certificate after death or within 14 days before death
- Unnatural deaths and accidents including:
  - road traffic accidents
  - domestic accidents
  - falls
  - fires.
- Death:
  - by violence
  - through neglect (including clinical negligence)
  - from abortion
  - in suspicious circumstances.
- Within 24 hours of operation or before recovery from anaesthetic
- Due to industrial disease
- Due to poisoning including:
  - drugs
  - alcohol.
- Criminal deaths:
  - murder
  - manslaughter
  - infanticide
  - assisted suicide.
- Suicides
- Infant deaths (including sudden infant deaths)

The completion of the Cremation Form generates a fee. Remember to keep a record of any cremation fees you receive for your tax return, unless the practice keeps the income generated.* If it is not paid immediately by the undertaker ask the appropriate member of practice staff to ensure the money is received.

* See Additional fees, p. 60.

Form C

This confirmatory medical certificate must be completed by a doctor who has been registered for at least 5 years. They must not be a partner or relative of the first doctor or the patient. Ideally they must examine the body and also see and question the doctor completing form B, but in practice this interview is often done over the phone. If you complete a form B expect a call from another doctor, usually another local GP. If a post-mortem has been done then the pathologist will sign this instead.

Supporting the bereaved

In supporting the recently bereaved with home visits and phone calls, some GPs prescribe temporary night sedation or diazepam to help them through the early days and funeral. Mark their medical records with the date of the bereavement so you can anticipate 'anniversary reactions'.

DRIVING

Many medical conditions and medications can affect driving and, although often overlooked in a busy surgery, it is a GP's duty to advise patients on their fitness to drive. Your essential reference is the *At a Glance Guide to the Current Medical Standards of Fitness to Drive* produced by the Driver and Vehicle Licensing Agency (DVLA). A copy should be available in your surgery.

GPs are also involved in assessing patients' fitness to hold driving licences and in completing medical assessment forms for parking for the disabled, seatbelt exemptions and eligibility for alternative transport schemes for the disabled.

As a GP registrar you may not have much direct involvement with such assessments and forms but it is useful to know what is involved for your future practice. Fitness to drive also often crops up in the MRCGP exam. Alcohol and driving are included for the sake of completeness.

Fitness to drive

> **Doctors must advise patients to notify the DVLA if they have a condition that affects their ability to drive. However it is the duty of the licence holder, and not the doctor, to inform the DVLA.**

Essentially anyone with a condition that might cause either a sudden or disabling event at the wheel, or affect the ability to control a vehicle safely, is not fit to drive. It is up to the DVLA to decide whether or not a patient is medically fit to drive so they need to be informed of relevant conditions. The *At a Glance Guide* is divided by medical condition for easy reference (*Box 24.5*) and you should familiarize yourself with the main stipulations.

You have a duty to ensure that your patient understands that their condition may impair their ability to drive and you should advise them that they are legally bound to inform the DVLA. If you forget to discuss it in the consultation then phone or write to the patient, particularly if there is a new diagnosis. Discuss the condition with the DVLA medical advisor if you are unsure whether it is relevant.

Following DVLA notification

Once the patient has notified the DVLA you may be contacted to provide a medical report. Check in the guide whether the patient is safe to drive pending the DVLA decision. You should also advise them to inform their motor insurance company and warn them that their insurance may be invalidated if they choose to ignore your advice.

For short periods of incapacity (i.e. up to 3 months) such as after surgery, drivers do not need to inform the DVLA, but there are some

---

Box 24.5 *At a glance guide*: medical categories

- Neurological disorders, particularly:
  - Epilepsy
  - Stroke
  - Dizzy spells.
- Cardiovascular disorders:
  - MI
  - angina
  - arrhythmias.
- Diabetes mellitus
- Psychiatric disorders
- Drug and alcohol misuse and dependency
- Visual disorders:
  - minimum visual acuity safe for driving.
- Renal, respiratory and sleep disorders
- Miscellaneous and elderly drivers:
  - pregnancy
  - main causes for concern in elderly.

---

neurological and cardiovascular exceptions to this. They will however need to inform their insurer. Arrange a review specifically to discuss returning to driving.

Patients often react badly to being told that they may need to give up driving. They may even disagree with the diagnosis or its effect on driving. If this is the case then suggest a second opinion (which you should arrange) and advise them not to drive in the meantime.

Patients refusing to disclose to the DVLA*

* Full GMC guidance in their booklet: *Confidentiality: protecting and providing information*: Appendix 2.

Occasionally a patient will tell you outright that they have no intention of stopping driving or will continue to drive against your advice. In such difficult cases you may need to breach patient confidentiality in order to protect their safety and that of others:

- if a patient is unable to understand that their condition affects their ability to drive (such as with dementia), then inform the DVLA immediately
- if a patient continues to drive when unfit then persuade them to stop. This may include involving their next of kin. If this is unsuccessful, or you are given evidence that they continue to drive, let the DVLA advisor know immediately.

If you do this you must inform the patient beforehand, that you intend to do so and afterwards, confirming that you have done so. Seek advice from your trainer in such cases.

Driving licences

The DVLA is responsible for issuing, renewing or withholding driving licences. There are two categories of licences and they have different health stipulations (*Box 24.6*).

GPs are involved in assessing fitness to drive for all HGV (group 2) licences and may be involved in confirming fitness in the over-70s with an ordinary licence. If you are required to undertake the odd medical for these familiarize yourself with the paperwork and clinical information required before launching into the examination. A fee is payable.

Driving and the elderly

You may need to persuade an elderly patient to give up driving on medical grounds. This is often received with a fear of loss of independence so encourage the use of other forms of transport. Some local authorities run schemes that give discounts on taxi fares. You may be asked to complete a medical form for these.

Quoted from *Grounds for Admission under the Mental Health Act 1983 England and Wales.* Crown copyright material is reproduced with the permission of the controller of HMSO and the Queen's Printer for Scotland.

Seatbelts

The driver and all front and back seat passengers must wear seatbelts, but there are a few exceptions. 'Certificates of Exemption from Compulsory Seatbelt Wearing' are available from Department of Health and need to be signed by a doctor.

Alcohol and driving

The legal limit of blood alcohol is 80 mg/100 ml blood, but it may be reduced to 50 mg/100 ml in future. There is great individual variation in alcohol metabolism so the oft-quoted statement that it takes 'one hour to clear a unit of alcohol' is not reliable.

THE MENTAL HEALTH ACT AND THE ACUTELY MENTALLY ILL PATIENT

The prospect of sectioning a patient in the community strikes fear into the hearts of most new GPs, particularly those who have not had experience as a psychiatry SHO. Although patients may need sectioning as inpatients (psychiatric or otherwise), here we only cover issues relating to patients in the community.

Only a small proportion of mentally ill patients will ever need to be detained under the Mental Health Act. Relatively few of these will be for the first presentation of an acute and violent psychosis. Sections can often be arranged at a relatively leisurely pace, as a situation deteriorates, in which case the mental health team can be mobilized in advance and assessments made at a mutually convenient time.

Although it can be quite obvious that a section is required, in other less clear-cut situations the decision will be shared between the GP, social worker and psychiatrist.

Make sectioning a tutorial topic and go through some section papers ('Medical Recommendation for Admission for Assessment' forms) before you need to use them in an emergency setting. Do your first section, at least, with your trainer. Truly urgent sections always seem to crop up on busy days and can feel pretty chaotic, but knowing who to contact can facilitate the process.

The Mental Health Act 1983 (England and Wales)

A patient with a mental disorder can be treated without their consent (i.e. compulsorily) for the mental disorder and severe physical disorder arising from that mental disorder. There are specific grounds for admission (*Box 24.7*) under the Act. Scotland and Northern Ireland have their own legislation: Mental Health (Scotland) Act 1984 and the Mental Health (Northern Ireland) Order 1986 which are similar, but not identical.

Box 24.7 Grounds for admission under the Mental Health Act 1983 (England and Wales)

- The patient suffers from a mental disorder of a nature or severity that justifies hospital admission

and

- admission is in the interests of the patient's own health and safety and/or the safety of others

and

- that voluntary admission is inappropriate – because the patient refuses admission or is unable to decide.

Inclusions and exclusions of the Act

Mental disorder includes mental illness (which is not actually defined in the Act), mental impairment (learning disability), psychopathic disorders and includes anorexia nervosa. It excludes drug and alcohol dependence, however mental disorder can co-exist with, or arise from, drug and alcohol use or withdrawal.

Where patients with physical disorders refuse consent to treatment they cannot be treated under the Act, unless the physical disorder arises from the mental disorder. In such cases, if the patient lacks the capacity to decide then the 'best interests' principle should be used.*

* See Treating incompetent adults: 'best interests' principle, p. 227.

Sections relevant to GPs

Only a few sections of the Act are relevant to GPs (*Box 24.8*). GPs should aim to use Section 2, which allows admission for 28 days. The emergency Section 4 should be avoided unless there would be a dangerous delay in transferring the patient to hospital whilst a second medical opinion is awaited. A Section 4 can be converted to a Section 2 or 3 once the patient is admitted.

Organizing a section

There are key personnel involved in arranging a mental health section and you will be assisting them, rather than taking responsibility for the section (*Box 24.9*). The Approved Social Worker (ASW) is the coordinator in the sectioning process and not the GP. Although CPNs are highly involved in the community mental health team, they do not actually have statutory involvement in sections. They may alert you when they feel one of their clients is deteriorating and may need a section.

The request for a mental health assessment, which may determine the need for a section, can come from a variety of sources:

- relatives, co-habitees and neighbours
- police or the ambulance service attending a violent patient
- ASW/CPN or other health professionals dealing with a patient.

The GP is often called in the first instance. Only a social worker or nearest relative can actually apply for the section. The GP and psychiatrist then make the recommendation for a section.

If a section seems likely do not panic! You will not have to deal with it alone. In some emergency cases the patient may have absconded by the time you get there, in which case the police and perhaps the police surgeon will have to deal with it.

Box 24.8

Box 24.8   Mental Health Act 1983 (England and Wales): sections relevant to general practice

Section 2 'Admission for Assessment'
- Application by a social worker or nearest relative (not neighbour)
- Requires medical assessment, recommendation and agreement by two doctors:
  - one Section 12-approved psychiatrist *and*
  - one who knows the patient (usually the GP).
- Allows for admission to hospital for assessment for 28 days. Treatment can also be given
- Diagnosis need not be clear
- Patient can be admitted within 14 days of the application
- Patient can appeal within first 14 days

Section 4 'Admission in an Emergency'
- Application as for Section 2
- Requires only one medical recommendation (preferably the GP but the doctor need not know the patient) in addition to the social worker
- Allows for admission for assessment for 72 hours only
- Patient should be admitted within 24 hours of the application or medical recommendation
- Should be reserved for 'emergency' situations when organizing a Section 2 would cause unnecessary delay
- Patient cannot appeal

Section 3 ' Admission for Treatment'
- Application, assessment and recommendation as for Section 2, but need for hospital treatment must be established
- Diagnosis must be known
- Patient may be admitted from community or more commonly already in hospital with Section 2 or 4
- Admission up to 6 months and renewable
- Patient can appeal during first 6 months

Before you go

Liaise with the duty Approved Social Worker who should arrange for the section to proceed safely and the relevant professionals to be available. They should arrange for the psychiatrist to meet you both at

Box 24.9   Key players in mental health assessments

Approved Social Worker (ASW)
- Key to the whole process
- May know the patient already
- Will have the relevant section papers
- Will do their own mental health assessment (MHA) on the patient
- Will find the Section 12-approved psychiatrist (below) for the assessment
- Have a statutory duty to inform the patient's family of the section
- May be able to locate a bed for the patient
- Keep contact number for duty ASW in your on-call paperwork

Section 12-approved psychiatrist
- Available on-call in the community
- Assesses patients to determine the need for a section in addition to the GP's opinion
- Receive a fee for this service
- Contactable via the ASW
- Will usually be the Responsible Medical Officer (RMO) taking overall responsibility for the section

---

the patient's address and they will have the relevant paperwork. Discuss the situation with your supervising GP colleague and ideally get them to come with you. Attend with an escort where possible. The police or ambulance service may also be at the scene.

Once there

You need to:

- put your own safety first. If you are confronted with an acutely disturbed patient retain a calm and reassuring air. They are often very frightened. Remain respectful and avoid anything that may provoke them. Ensure you remain between the patient and the nearest exit*
- decide if hospital admission is needed
- try to persuade them to agree voluntarily if possible
- establish whether there are grounds for admission under the Mental Health Act, if they refuse.

* See also Safety matters, p. 78 and Defusing a potentially violent situation, p. 90.

After the assessment

Once you have made your assessment and recommended a section then complete and sign the papers and leave them with the social worker. Unless the patient needs acute medical treatment, such as sedation, you can then go. Document fully your assessment and reasoning for use of the Mental Health Act in the medical record. Debrief later with your trainer.

If a section is not needed

Arrange alternative management such as medication, voluntary admission or outpatient review with increased input from the CPN and/or social services in the meantime.

Other situations

It may become apparent on a routine home visit that a full mental health assessment is needed, in which case it is reasonable to go back to your surgery and contact the mental health team from there. When the social worker and Section 12 doctor have made their assessment, ask them to liaise with you at the surgery to complete the section papers rather than return to the patient, particularly if they are acutely disturbed.

You may be asked to attend a psychiatric ward to assess one of your own patients admitted under Section 2 in order to convert this to a Section 3 for treatment. You should try to discuss the case with the psychiatric consultant (or one of the team) and social worker before making your assessment and signing the paperwork.

Appeals against sections

Patients and nearest relatives can appeal to have sections revoked by application to a Mental Health Review Tribunal which consists of a psychiatrist, lawyer and a lay member. The Mental Health Act Commission, a special health authority that oversees the operation of the Mental Health Act, also investigates complaints made by detained patients.

Discharge

The hospital should always let you know directly when a sectioned patient is discharged. A multidisciplinary pre-discharge meeting is arranged (under the Care Programme Approach) with details of all the professionals involved, treatment requirements and dates for review team meetings. A key-worker is allocated to coordinate the care plan and ensure communication across the professionals.

NOTIFIABLE DISEASES

Under the Public Health (Control of Disease) Act 1984 and Public Health (Infectious Diseases) Regulations 1988 doctors are obliged to notify the 'relevant local authority officer' of the identity and address of any person suspected of having a notifiable disease (*Box 24.10*) or food poisoning. If in doubt discuss the case with your local Public Health Department. There are some variations in the list of notifiable diseases in Scotland and Northern Ireland.

It is uncommon to notify diseases in routine general practice and most notifications will be for food poisoning. Microbiology labs will often prompt you to notify by a comment on the pathology report. AIDS is not a notifiable disease, but a voluntary confidential reporting scheme exists provided the patient agrees.

Your practice will have a book of notification forms for completion together with the local forwarding address to the Medical Officer for Environmental Health. A small fee is payable. Always inform any patients you notify and tell them why. Warn them that they may be contacted by Public Health Department staff, particularly if they are food-handlers.

Box 24.10   Notifiable diseases

Anthrax	Paratyphoid fever A and B
Cholera	Plague
Diphtheria	Polio
Dysentery (amoebic, bacillary)	Rabies
Ebola virus disease	Relapsing fever
Encephalitis	Rubella
Food poisoning (any)	Scarlet fever
Lassa fever	Smallpox
Leprosy	Tetanus
Leptospirosis	Tuberculosis
Malaria	Typhoid fever
Marburg disease	Typhus fever
Measles	Viral haemorrhagic fever
Meningitis	Viral hepatitis
Meningococcal sepsis	Whooping cough
Mumps	Yellow fever
Ophthalmia neonatorum	

Quoted from form HSA1. Crown copyright material is reproduced with the permission of the controller of HMSO and the Queen's Printer for Scotland.

POWER OF ATTORNEY

This legal document allows someone to pass over control of their financial affairs and property to another (the attorney) and is particularly relevant in the management of patients with dementia.

Ordinary power of attorney is appropriate where someone (the donor) needs another person to manage their affairs temporarily, but this power is invalidated if the donor becomes mentally incapacitated (i.e. legally incompetent). An enduring power of attorney continues even if the donor becomes mentally incapacitated. It is important to consider this in the early stages of dementia as the donor must have sufficient competence to grant the power in the first place.

GPs may be asked to comment on a patient's capacity to agree to setting one up, but it may be prudent to get another specialist opinion (e.g. from a psychogeriatrician). There are specific guidelines on assessing mental capacity from the BMA in conjunction with the Law Society.*

* See Sources and further reading.

Advise anyone applying for this (usually a relative) to contact a Citizens' Advice Bureau, solicitor or law centre to ensure all the legal formalities involved are complied with.

TERMINATION OF PREGNANCY

All GPs will come across requests for terminations (TOPs). If you have conscientious or religious objections you are not obliged to treat the woman or sign the paperwork. You do, however, have a duty to refer her promptly to another doctor who is willing to counsel and refer as needed, which will usually be one of your GP colleagues. If you are not prepared to organize TOPs for patients, make it clear to your trainer at the beginning of the year so arrangements can be made for another doctor to see such patients with minimum inconvenience.

The Abortion Act 1967 and The Human Fertilization and Embryology Act 1990

These Acts allow a termination of pregnancy to be carried out legally in the circumstances specified on an HSA1 form, 'Certificate A' (*Box 24.11*). A termination can be carried out at *any* gestation if there is a substantial risk that the child would be seriously handicapped or the mother's life or health is in grave danger. Other criteria allow for a termination up to the end of the 24th week of pregnancy. Most termination requests in general practice will be satisfied by the criteria in section C even if there is no obvious or immediate threat to the woman's mental or physical health.

Box 24.11   Criteria for a legal termination of pregnancy

A The continuance of the pregnancy would involve risk to the life of the pregnant woman greater than if the pregnancy were terminated

B The termination is necessary to prevent grave permanent injury to the physical or mental health of the pregnant woman

C The pregnancy has not exceeded its 24th week and the continuance of the pregnancy would involve risk, greater than if the pregnancy were terminated, of injury to the physical or mental health of the pregnant woman

D The pregnancy has not exceeded its 24th week and the continuance of the pregnancy would involve risk, greater than if the pregnancy were terminated, of injury to the physical or mental health of any existing child(ren) of the family of the pregnant woman

E There is a substantial risk that if the child were born it would suffer from such physical or mental abnormalities as to be seriously handicapped

Reproduced from form HSA1.

The HSA1 form must be completed and signed by two doctors who have seen the woman, but it is not necessary for both to examine the woman. The GP is usually the first signatory and the form is then to be sent with the referral to the TOP clinic for the clinic or hospital doctor to complete it.

A further form is sent to the 'Chief Officer of the Minister of Health' by the doctor undertaking the procedure within 7 days, confirming that the termination has been carried out.

All terminations must be carried out in approved hospitals, including some private clinics. Most regions offer an NHS-based termination service through the hospital or community gynaecology service, but may contract this out to a local private or charity service.

Arranging NHS terminations

Find out how best to refer locally and what the clinic will undertake (including medical terminations). In some regions women may arrange a clinic appointment themselves through a central booking service, but they still require a GP referral letter. Have this appointments number to hand in your surgery. Otherwise your practice secretary or receptionist should arrange the appointment by phone and the woman should be advised to return in a few days to collect their referral letter, HSA1 form and appointment time.

Advise women they will not have the actual termination on the day of their clinic appointment.

Where dates are uncertain or the woman presents late you may wish to arrange an urgent dating ultrasound, or refer them urgently so the clinic can do this.

Clinics usually request the cover of GP out-of-hours services for day case procedures.

Private clinics

Several private and voluntary sector agencies offer pregnancy counselling and terminations. Charges are around £300–400 and women may self-refer. This may be an option for those who can afford it and cannot tolerate the wait on the NHS.

Well-known organizations include the Brook Advisory Service, British Pregnancy Advisory Service and Marie Stopes Clinics; details are in the phone directories.

SOURCES AND FURTHER READING

General

1. Knight B. *Legal Aspects of Medical Practice*, 5th edn. Churchill Livingstone, 1992.
2. Sandell A. *Oxford Handbook of Patients' Welfare.* Oxford, 1998.
3. Marquand P. *Introduction to Medical Law.* Butterworth Heinemann, 2000.
4. Palmer K.T. *Notes for the MRCGP*, 3rd edn. Blackwell Science, 1998.

Advance directives

5. BMA Code of Practice and Guidance on Advance Statements, 1995.
6. Medical Protection Society. *Managing the Risks in General Practice.* MPS, 2001.
7. The Terrence Higgins Trust, 52–54 Grays Inn Road, London WC1X 8JU; Tel: 0845 122 1200; website, www.tht.org.uk
8. Voluntary Euthanasia Society, 13 Prince of Wales Terrace, London W8 5PG.

Child protection

9. Department of Health. *Child Protection; Medical Responsibilities*, 1994.
10. National Society for the Prevention of Cruelty to Children website www.nspcc.org.uk

Deaths

13. Death and cremation certificates.
14. Benefits Agency booklet D49, *What to do after a Death in England and Wales*. April 2000.

Driving

15. DVLA website www.dvla.gov.uk
16. DVLA. *At a Glance Guide to the Current Medical Standards of Fitness to Drive*, August 2001.
17. GMC. *Confidentiality: protecting and providing information*. GMC, September 2000.

Mental health

18. Section papers.
19. Bradley J.J. *The Mental Health Act 1983 (England and Wales), Mental Health (Patients in the Community) Act 1995*. Medical Protection Society, 1997.
20. GMC. *Seeking patients' consent, the ethical considerations*: GMC, November 1998.

Notifiable diseases

21. Notification certificates.
22. Montgomery J. *Health Care Law*. Oxford University Press, 1997.

Power of attorney

23. BMA and The Law Society. *Assessment of Mental Capacity: Guidance for Doctors and Lawyers*, 1995.

Termination of pregnancy

24. HSA1 form.

25

Options at the end of the year

INTRODUCTION

> **You must have your JCPTGP certificate in order to work as a GP in the UK. Ensure you have applied for your certificate within the last month of your registrar year.**

The majority of newly qualified GPs do not follow the direct path from registrar to partner. Aside from locum work there are numerous opportunities and GPs are in a great position to work flexibly, in different posts and with control over their working hours and conditions. General practice has been described as the 'original portfolio career' and armed with your JCPTGP certificate and, even better, the MRCGP exam, you can consider a wide variety of career options from journalism to occupational health. You could combine a community health job with GP sessions, or move into research for a year or two.

WORKING AS A NON-PRINCIPAL

Non-principals are required to register with a health authority in order to work in general practice in a given area. Send them your curriculum vitae with a couple of references to ensure inclusion on their list of non-principals.

Join, or set up, a non-principals group so you can share ideas, job information and keep up-to-date with clinical issues. Join the National Association of Non-Principals.*

* See p. 42.

Locums

Locum work may be particularly convenient if you are working for the MRCGP exam after completing your registrar year. Working as a GP locum is an excellent way to see how other practices operate and gain experience of different patient groups. Organization, workload and ethos vary enormously between practices. Working in different settings can give you clear ideas about what you do and do not want when, and if, you commit to a permanent post.

You need to have all your own equipment so restock your bag. You may have to buy your drug supplies on a private prescription. Make sure your medical protection organization and GMC subscriptions are up-to-date. You should also have confirmation of your hepatitis B immunity status for employers.

Getting work

Organize yourself before the end of the registrar year to avoid a break in earnings (*Box 25.1*).

Box 25.1   Finding locum work

- Get a list of all local practices from the health authority
- Update your curriculum vitae and circulate it to local practices with a covering letter to the practice manager
- Let your training practice know you are looking for work and notify other GPs through the cooperative or your VTS colleagues
- Register with local locum groups or agencies
- Put up a notice at the local cooperative if they are agreeable
- Look for adverts in the *BMJ Careers* and the GP press
- Ensure you have a mobile phone, diary and a system to avoid double booking

---

Money matters

Locums are self-employed so you will need a system to produce invoices, keep receipts and track of your accounts. You will be responsible for paying your own tax so keep money aside (approximately a third) for this. Put this in a high-interest, easy-access savings account. Discuss your financial status with a small business advisor at your bank and an accountant. You will need to register to pay class 2 (self-employed) National Insurance contributions with the Inland Revenue NI contributions office. You can claim work-related expenses against tax (telephone, stationery, travel expenses, etc.) so keep all receipts carefully filed. Consider keeping a spreadsheet of your income and outgoings as you go. It is a good idea to have a separate bank account or credit card for work-related costs.

Confirm or negotiate fees before you commit to a locum and establish whether you will be paid an hourly, sessional or all-day rate. Clarify whether visits or on-call duties are included and, if not, charge extra. Invoice practices at the time of the session or soon afterwards and keep a record of unpaid sessions so you can remind practice managers.

Your pay will be irregular so you may need a 'cushion' or reasonable overdraft facility to ensure your regular bills are covered. You will miss out on holiday, sick and maternity pay and paid study leave, so take this into account when deciding how much you need to work and earn.

Non-principals are entitled to contribute to the NHS pension scheme, so keep accurate details of your locum earnings, for whom you worked and when.

Support

It is common to feel somewhat under-confident immediately after training so work in larger practices initially and avoid isolated single-handed practices. Let the practice know that you have recently completed your training and confirm that other doctors will be working at the same time. Do not hesitate to ask for clinical advice.

Practices should provide you with a locum pack including the main paperwork you need, practice telephone numbers, prescribing policy and referral information.

Although you may be anxious about getting work initially, take care not to overbook yourself or neglect regular breaks. The locum lifestyle can be chaotic, which is tiring in itself.

GP assistants and salaried GPs

PCGs and PCTs, PMS projects and individual practices offer a number of different types of salaried and assistant posts. Practices with a particularly large list size may apply for health authority reimbursement for such posts.

These posts may offer clinical sessions in a practice with sessions in another specialty or in research and can be ideal for newly qualified GPs. They may include protected time for peer support, audit and practice development.

Salaries vary around the country and contracts are usually for 12–24 months. Ensure you have a contract and are adequately remunerated for on-call work. Stipulations for holidays, sick pay and pension contributions should be clear. You should have the option for a 3-month review of your workload and salary. If you are employed by a practice you may need to negotiate your pay.

Check the *BMJ Careers* section for adverts.

Retainer scheme

Under this scheme, GPs with outside commitments who cannot work full-time, can work regularly on a part-time basis. Retainer GPs are employed by a practice to work between one and four sessions a week for up to 5 years, although extensions are possible.

This scheme is typically used by women with young families who wish to 'keep their hand in', but other outside interests can also qualify. The health authority reimburses part of the salary and the retainer must justify why they can only work a few sessions a week. They must have long-term plans to return to general practice more fully in the future.

The practice has a responsibility to provide a named partner to support and train the retainer, who in turn must show evidence of on-going learning. The retainer is employed by the practice and has full employee benefits.

PARTNERSHIP

The big step – finally getting your name on the stationery! Many GPs still see partnership as the ultimate goal, but deciding when and where can be problematic. It is increasingly common for GPs to move around and change partnerships so it need not be viewed as a life-long commitment.

Getting to know patients, families and communities long-term can be very rewarding. Deciding how you work and developing your practice and services can be very stimulating. There is also the benefit of permanence, job security and usually increased income.

Doing your research

Choosing a partnership is a complicated business, so take your time to research it fully. Before agreeing to a position spend time with each partner and the practice manager, and ask the opinion of local doctors.

Time spent as a locum is an excellent way to see the day-to-day running of the practice. No practice is perfect but it is better to know the personalities and potential problems before you start. If you are keen on a place but not absolutely sure then ask to work for 6–12 months in a salaried capacity before you commit more fully. Otherwise consider an opt-out clause in your agreement after 3–6 months of working as a partner.

Financial matters

You must know what the situation is regarding remuneration. Do not be afraid to ask to see the practice accounts and practice agreement.

Remember that principals are self-employed and their income is generated by the business work of the practice. How they divide it between partners is another matter. You need to consider the following questions:

- If the premises are owned, are you expected to buy in?
- Will you start on less than full parity? If so, when will you reach full parity?
- Are profits distributed equally?
- What about medical income earned outside the practice?
- Is the practice GMS or PMS?

With recruitment difficulties in many parts of the UK a new partner is often in an excellent position to negotiate full parity and a delay before contributing to practice assets.

Salaried partners

These increasingly prevalent posts are a good option for doctors who want security and permanence without all the management and financial commitments of full partnership. There is an obvious overlap between such posts and salaried GPs and assistants.

Your contract should specify leave, sick pay and pension. Retain the option to re-negotiate your terms of employment at 3 months and a year.

ACADEMIC POSTS

Primary care is a growing academic discipline and there are often full- or part-time lecturer, researcher and other posts available at your local academic Department of General Practice or Primary Care. All have websites and it is worth checking out their main research interests, recent grant awards and publications, before applying for a post.

Funding is available for individual research work from RCGP fellowships and other grants and charities. Research general practices exist around the country with special funding.

Working for a higher degree in primary care (MSc or PhD) will provide a good basis for continuing with sessional research work throughout your career.

Academic departments organize student teaching and they may offer opportunities for undergraduate teaching in general practice. Jobs are usually advertised in the *BMJ*, otherwise enquire at your local department. Remuneration may be less than for clinical posts.

OTHER SESSIONAL WORK

There are many opportunities to work as a GP on a sessional basis for NHS and other organizations (*Box 25.2*). As with academic

Box 25.2   Opportunities for sessional work

NHS
- Out-of-hours cooperatives
- Family planning
- Pregnancy advisory services
- Genitourinary medicine
- Homeless projects
- Drug and alcohol services
- NHS walk-in centres

Private
- Deputizing services
- Private screening medicals (e.g. for BUPA)
- Slimming clinics
- Drug rehabilitation units
- Medical support for events
- Private general practice

medicine this can be on a regular or *ad hoc* basis. Posts may be advertised in the *BMJ*, otherwise ask around locally or contact the organizations themselves.

OTHER CAREERS AND QUALIFICATIONS

GPs are in a good position to look at careers outside general practice (*Box 25.3*). These can be pursued full-time or alongside general practice on a part-time or sessional basis.

Consider qualifications in addition to the MRCGP exam to stimulate interest and to make you more employable.

WORKING ABROAD

Always clarify qualification, work permit and visa requirements.

Once you've completed your GP training, you may feel it is an excellent time to consider a spell working abroad. Your training will be recognized in all European Community countries. Although language may be a barrier, there are some English-speaking posts abroad. Medical French and Spanish courses are occasionally advertised in the *BMJ*.

Australia and New Zealand offer GP posts to UK-trained doctors, usually in areas where they have found difficulty in recruiting.

Voluntary organizations such as Voluntary Services Overseas (VSO), International Health Exchange and Médecins Sans Frontières can arrange placements in developing countries or war-torn areas. They may require a relatively long-term commitment. Working as a ship's doctor is also an option if you have sea legs.

BACK TO HOSPITAL

Returning to a 6-month SHO post, or career-grade post, may be an option. Your GP registrar year may have highlighted areas in which you would benefit from more training, or have simply stimulated a clinical interest.

This can also be useful for women planning a family and hoping to avoid a break in NHS service.

SOURCES AND FURTHER READING

1. Chambers R., Mohanna K., Field S. *Options and Opportunities in Medical Careers.* Radcliffe Medical Press, 2000.
2. Hastie A. *The General Practice Retainer Scheme. BMJ Career Focus,* 21 July 2001.

3. O'Connell S. *Handbook for Non-Principals in General Practice*, NANP
   Limited Edition Press 1998, and also available on National Association of
   Non-Principals website, www.nanp.org.uk
4. Faculty of Occupational Health website, www.faoccmed.ac.uk
5. The National Sports Medicine Institute of the UK website,
   www.nsmi.org.uk
6. Faculty of Public Health Medicine website, www.fphm.org.uk
7. Faculty of Pharmaceutical Medicine website, www.fpm.org.uk
8. Association of Police Surgeons website, www.apsweb.org.uk
9. Royal College of Physicians (London) website, www.rcplondon.ac.uk
10. British Society of Rehabilitation Medicine website, www.bsrm.co.uk
11. Voluntary Service Overseas website, www.vso.org.uk
12 International Health Exchange website, www.ihe.org.uk
13. Médecins Sans Frontières website, www.msf.org.uk

General practice forms

DS 1500	Application form for benefits, including DLA and AA for terminally ill patients with a prognosis of less than 6 months
D4	Application and medical report form for Group 2 driving licences
FP7 & 8	GP medical record continuation cards
FP10	Standard GP prescription form
FP10 Comp	Computer prescription form
FP10 MDA	Prescription form for prescribing in treatment of addiction
FP92A	Application form for exemption from prescription charges for medical reasons
FW8	Application form for exemption from prescription charges for maternity reasons
GMS 1–4	Health authority forms for claiming fees for patient services undertaken
GOS18	Request for ophthalmology opinion from optician to GP
GP10	Prescription form (Scotland)
HC2	Certificate for full exemption from NHS health charges
HSA1	Termination of Pregnancy form
IB113	Medical form for completion prior to a Personal Capability Assessment
MAT B1	Form for claiming maternity benefits
Med 3–6	Statutory sickness certificates
RM7	Form to request a Personal Capability Assessment where incapacity/illness is in doubt
SC1 and 2	Self-certificate forms to claim sickness pay
VTR/1 and 2	Statements of satisfactory completion of either GP registrar post or educationally approved posts for GP training

Useful addresses & websites

We have included addresses and websites that were useful in researching this book and we do not claim to be comprehensive. Addresses do change so use the links on larger websites and check for updates on our BIOS website.

Some sites are in the public domain and others restrict access to doctors or registered users.

TRAINING AND EDUCATION

The Joint Committee on Postgraduate Training for General Practice (JCPTGP)
www.jcptgp.org.uk

> 14 Princes Gate
> Hyde Park
> London SW7 1PU
> **Tel 020 7581 3232**
> **Fax 020 7589 5047**

Royal College of General Practitioners (RCGP)
www.rcgp.org.uk

> 14 Princes Gate
> Hyde Park
> London SW7 1PU
> **Tel 020 7581 3232**
> **Fax 020 7225 3047**

National Office for Summative Assessment
www.doctoronline.nhs.uk

> King Alfred's College
> Winchester
> Hants
> SO22 4NR
> **Tel 01962 827389**
> **Fax 01962 827437**

Royal College of Obstetricians and Gynaecologists
www.rcog.org.uk

27 Sussex Place
Regents Park
London NW1 4RG
Tel 020 7772 6200

Faculty of Family Planning and Reproductive Healthcare of the RCOG
www.ffprhc.org.uk

19 Cornwall Terrace
London NW1 4QP
Tel 020 7935 7149

Royal College of Paediatrics and Child Health
www.rcpch.ac.uk

50 Hallam Street
London W1W 6DE
Tel 020 7307 5600

Royal College of Physicians of London
www.rcplondon.ac.uk

11 St Andrew's Place
Regents Park
London NW1 4LE
Tel 020 7935 1174

Conference of Postgraduate Medical Deans in the UK
www.copmed.org.uk

Royal Society of Medicine
www.roysocmed.ac.uk

1 Wimpole Street
London W1G OAE
Tel 020 7290 2900

www.doctors.net.uk
Medical website available to GMC registered doctors with on-line textbooks, Medline, Cochrane Database, access to poisons information database and Travax (travel medicine database).

GENERAL PROFESSIONAL

General Medical Council
www.gmc-uk.org

178 Great Portland Street
London W1N 6JE
Tel 020 7580 7642

British Medical Association
www.bma.org.uk

BMA House
Tavistock Square
London WC1H 9JK
Tel 020 7387 4499

General Practitioners Committee
www.bma.org.uk/gpc.nsf

British Medical Journal
www.bmj.com

BMJ Careers
www.bmjcareers.com

BMJ Bookshop
www.bmjbookshop.com

Burton Street
London WC1H 9JR
Tel 020 7383 6244

Medical Protection Society
www.mps.org.uk

Granary Wharf House
Leeds LS11 5PY
and
33 Cavendish Square
London W1G 0PS
Membership Tel 0845 718 7187
and
Medico-legal help 0845 605 4000

The Medical Defence Union
www.the-mdu.com

230 Blackfriars Road
London SE1 8PJ
and

7 Cope Street
Dublin 2
Advisory help-line 0800 716646
Press office 020 7202 1535

National Association of Non-Principals
www.nanp.org.uk.

PO Box 188
Chichester
West Sussex
PO19 2ZA
Fax 01243 536428 (no phone)

National Association of GP Co-operatives
www.nagpc.org.uk

HEALTH SERVICE

The National Health Service
www.nhs.uk

Department of Health
www.doh.gov.uk

Health of Wales Information Service
www.wales.nhs.uk

Department of Health, Social Services and Public Safety in Northern
Ireland
www.dhsspsni.gov.uk

Scottish Executive Health Department in Scotland
www.show.scot.nhs.uk

National Institute of Clinical Excellence
www.nice.org.uk

Commission for Health Improvement
www.chi.nhs.uk

National Patient Safety Agency
www.npsa.org.uk

Health and Safety Executive
www.hse.gov.uk

Department for Work and Pensions
www.dwp.gov.uk

NHS Zero Tolerance Zone Campaign
www.nhs.uk/zerotolerance

UK National Screening Committee
www.doh.gov.uk/nsc/index.htm

PRESCRIBING

British National Formulary
www.BNF.org

Drug and Therapeutics Bulletin
www.which.net/health/dtb/

National Prescribing Centre
www.npc.co.uk

Medicines Control Agency
www.open.gov.uk/mca/mcahome.htm

Prescription Pricing Authority
www.ppa.org.uk

PATIENT-RELEVANT

Driver and Vehicle Licensing Agency (DVLA)
www.dvla.gov.uk

Drivers' Medical Unit
Longview Road
Morriston
Swansea SA99 ITU
Tel 01792 783686
and
Driver and Vehicle Licensing Northern Ireland
Castlerock Road
Coleraine BT51 3HS
Tel 01265 41200

The Aviation Health Institute
www.aviation-health.org

NHS A to Z Help-Direct website
www.nhsatoz.org

NHS Direct website
www.nhsdirect.nhs.uk

National Society for the Prevention of Cruelty to Children
www.nspcc.org.uk

Citizens' Advice Bureau
www.nacab.org.uk

OTHER RELATED CAREERS

Faculty of Occupational Health
www.facoccmed.ac.uk

Faculty of Public Health Medicine
www.fphm.org.uk

Faculty of Pharmaceutical Medicine
www.fpm.org.uk

The National Sports Medicine Institute of the UK
www.nsmi.org.uk

Association of Police Surgeons
www.apsweb.org.uk

British Society of Rehabilitation Medicine
www.bsrm.co.uk

OVERSEAS VOLUNTARY WORK

Voluntary Service Overseas (VSO)
www.vso.org.uk

International Health Exchange
www.ihe.org.uk

Médecins Sans Frontières
www.msf.org.uk

Recommended reading

Personal preference, familiarity and recommendations from friends and colleagues are usually the basis of any personal library. We have included some suggestions here for the basic GP books you need to read or dip in to. We have purposefully kept the list brief and it should be considered your minimum requirements.

Many of these are regularly updated so always refer to the latest edition. Some are available on-line.

REFERENCE TEXTS

British National Formulary 42, British Medical Association and Royal Pharmaceutical Society of Great Britain, 2001.

Barton S.W., *Clinical Evidence*, Issue 5, BMJ Publishing Group, 2001.

Hope R.A., Longmore J.M., McManus S.K., Wood-Allum C.A., *Oxford Handbook of Clinical Medicine*, 4th edition, Oxford University Press, 1998.

Collier J.A.B., Longmore J.M., Brown T.J., *Oxford Handbook of Clinical Specialties*, 5th edition, Oxford University Press, 1999.

Sandell A., *Oxford Handbook of Patients' Welfare*, Oxford University Press, 1998.

OTC (Over the Counter) Directory, Proprietary Association of Great Britain.

The Department of Health, *Immunisation Against Infectious Diseases*, HMSO, 1996.

The Department of Health, *Health Information for Overseas Travel*, HMSO, 2000.

At a Glance Guide to the Current Medical Standards of Fitness to Drive, DVLA 2001.

GENERAL PRACTICE TEXTS

Schroeder K., *Top Tips for GPs*, Radcliffe Medical Press, 2001.

Khot A. and Polmear A., *Practical General Practice*, 3rd Edition, Butterworth-Heinemann, 1999.

Cartwright S. and Godlee, C.J., *Churchill's Pocket Book of General Practice*, Churchill Livingstone, 1998.

O'Connell S., *Handbook for Non-Principals in General Practice*, The Limited Edition Press, 1998.

CONSULTATION TEXTS

Neighbour R., *The Inner Consultation*, Petroc Press, 1999.

Pendleton D. *et al. The Consultation*, Oxford University Press, 1984.

Tate P., *The Doctor's Communication Handbook*, 3rd Edition, Radcliffe Medical Press, 2001.

Balint M., *The Doctor, His Patient and the Illness*, Churchill Livingstone, 2000.

MRCGP EXAM TEXTS

Palmer K.T., *Notes for the MRCGP*, 3rd Edition, Blackwell Science, 1998.

Stacey E., *Hot Topics in General Practice*, 3rd Edition, BIOS Scientific Publishers, 2000.

Stacey E. and Toun Y., *Critical Reading Questions for the MRCGP*, BIOS Scientific Publishers, 1997.

Kilburn J., *Answer Plans for the MRCGP*, BIOS Scientific Publishers, 2000.

Greenhalgh T., *How to Read a Paper*, 2nd Edition, BMJ Publishing Group, 2000.

Coggon D., *Statistics in Clinical Practice*, BMJ Publishing Group, 1995.

Ridsdale L., *Evidence-based General Practice*, WB Saunders, 1995.

PRACTICE MANAGEMENT

Ellis N., Chisholm J. and Bogle I., *Making Sense of the Red Book*, 3rd Edition, Radcliffe Medical Press, 1997.

Index

Fitness to work, **149–151**
Flatterers, 91
Flexible (part-time) training, 5
Follow up, 83, **84–85,** 87, 89–90, 131,
    136–9,141–3, 173, 180–181
Food poisoning, notifying, 256
Form-filling, **158–159**
FP7, 72, 271
FP8, 72, 271
FP92A (*see* Medical exemption certificate)
FP10, 97, 98, 271
FP10 comp, 97, 121, 271
FP10 MDA, 107, 271
FRCGP (Fellowship of the Royal College of
    General Practitioners), 43
Frequent attenders, 93
Friends and family, as patients, 94
Funeral directors, 244
FW8 (*see* Maternity exemption certificate)

General Medical Council, **38**
General Medical Services (GMS), 16–17
    Terms of Service, 18 (box 2.2), 159
General Practitioners Committee (GPC), 3, **41**
    GP Registrars' Subcommittee, **41–42**
    GP Registrars' Subcommittee, registrars'
        pack, 46 (box 5.1), 54
Generic prescribing (*see* Prescribing, generic)
Gifts from patients, **93–94**
Gillick competence, (*see* Competence, under
    16's and Consent, under 16's)
GMS (*see* General Medical Services)
GMS forms 1–4, 72, 271
Good prescribing practice, (*see* Prescribing,
    good practice)
GOS 18, 35, 271
GP Assistant (*see* Non-principal GP, assistant)
GP Associate (*see* Non-principal GP, associate)
GP cooperatives (*see* Cooperatives)
GP registrars' annual conference, 189
GP trainer, (*see also* Summative Assessment,
    Structured Trainer's Report) 3 (box 1.1),
    76–77, 186
    making the most of, 186
    problems with, 186
GP trainers, requirements, 10 (box 1.4), 55
    (box 6.1)
GP training, application, **6 – 9**
    application, choosing your practice, 9, 11
        (box 1.5)
    application, looking for jobs, 6–7
    application, non-UK nationals, 6
    application, the registrar year, 9
    organisation, **4–6**
    requirements, **2–4**
    requirements, approved (listed) specialties,
        2, **4** (box 1.2),
GP, principal (*see* Principal GP)
GP10, 107, 271
Guidelines, 87, 150, 161

HC2 charges certificate, 108, 271
Health and safety, (*see also* Safety, personal)
    48 (box 5.3),
    computers, 120
    consultation room, 69
    dispensing medicines, 69
    specimens, 139 (box 13.3)
Health authority lists, 190, **191**
Health promotion, 85, **87**
Health visitors, **29–30,** 240 (box 24.1)
Heartsinks, **92** (box 9.2)
Hidden agenda, 86, 88, 140, 150
Hidden consultations (*see* Consultations,
    hidden)
High-cost medication, 111
Holiday cancellation, letters, 161
Home visits, 29, 51, 166, **169–173**
    alternatives to, 171–172, 178
    an approach to **171–173**
    asking for help, 172
    daytime, 171
    if there is no answer, 172
    negotiating **181**
    practical preparations, 64–69, **170**
    safety precautions, **170** (box 17.1), 172
    transport, 170
    urgent, 164, 171
Homeopathic treatment (*see* Complementary
    medicine)
Hospital colleagues (*see* Asking for help and
    Referrals)
Hospital jobs, **7– 8**
    approval of posts/JCPTGP standards, 7–8
        (box 1.3)
    making the most of, 8
    vocational training statements, 7, 14
Hospital outpatients, sitting in, 189
Hot topics, (*see* MRCGP exam, hot topics)
Housebound patients, elderly, 173
    investigations (*see* Investigations,
        housebound patients)
Housing letters, 160
HSA1 form (*see* Termination of pregnancy,
    HSA1 form)
Human Fertilization and Embryology Act
    1990, The, 257–258
Hybrid schemes (*see* Innovative schemes)

IB113 form, 150, 271
Inappropriate patient requests, 89
Incapacity Benefit, 149, 152 (box 14.3)
Income Support, 152 (box 14.3)
Income, general practitioner, **19–21**
    general practitioner, NHS, 19 (box 2.3), 176
    general practitioner, non-NHS, 20 (box
        2.4), 56, 60, 159
Induction period, GP registrar, **46–49**
Informed consent, (*see* Consent, informed)
Innovative (hybrid) schemes, 5
Internet (*see also* e-Mail), 122